The Healing P

"There are many healing elements available in us and around us and it is possible to make use of them right away. Dr. Gabriel S. Weiss shows us in this book how to do so. He is a skilled practitioner of medicine and meditation. He has practiced meditation with us at Deer Park Monastery for several years and has a beautiful dharma name: Compassionate Service of the Heart. Enjoy this wonderful book and allow it to water the seeds of wisdom and compassion in you, which will bring healing and happiness to you and your beloved ones."

—THICH NHAT HANH, ZEN MASTER

"Our shelves are filled with useful perspectives on meditation, but as a physician attempting to help others make practical use of this growing literature, it is clear that *The Healing Power of Meditation* fills a true need. No other contribution brings together specific medical problems with pragmatic instruction, while also showing us how the meditative, contemplative, and scientific traditions share a common biological basis."

—THOMAS J. CHIPPENDALE, M.D., PH.D., PRACTICING NEUROLOGIST; MEDICAL DIRECTOR OF THE NEUROSCIENCES AND STROKE PROGRAMS FOR SCRIPPS HOSPITAL, ENCINITAS, CALIFORNIA; PRESIDENT, SAN DIEGO STROKE COUNCIL; AND TEACHER, MINDFULNESS-BASED STRESS REDUCTION

"In his book, Dr. Gabriel Weiss, whom I have known for many years, gives a very descriptive and practical approach to meditation. I will be recommending this book as an important tool to be used in the healing process of patients and to anyone who wishes to decrease stress and anxiety in their daily life."

—DANIEL VICARIO, M.D., MEDICAL ONCOLOGIST; CO-FOUNDER, SAN DIEGO CANCER CENTER (SDCC); AND DIRECTOR, SDCC INTEGRATIVE MEDICINE PROGRAM

"The Healing Power of Meditation is more than a book about meditation. It is a practical, understandable, comprehensive guide for a philosophy of life that bridges current Western and ancient Eastern Zen concepts. Dr. Weiss illustrates his principles with examples from his personal life and practice, and offers tips on implementing proposed exercises. The book also summarizes well the scientific evidence showing a benefit for using meditation to treat or prevent many illnesses, including diseases affected by the immune system such as asthma, infection, and cancer. Whether you are challenged medically, emotionally, or spiritually, or whether you just want to be a whole person, this book and its accompanying CD will enhance your life."

—RICHARD T. WOLD, M.D., GRADUATE, STANFORD MEDICAL SCHOOL; SPECIALIST IN ARTHRITIS AND ALLERGY; BOARD-CERTIFIED ALLERGIST AND CLINICAL IMMUNOLOGIST

"Dr. Weiss provides a valuable introduction to the vital importance of the relationship between mind and body in the healing process. He has collected and digested the relevant research of others and blended it with his own insights, moving stories and his years of experience and medical training. To this he has added a skillful and pragmatic presentation of the ancient wisdom and benefits of mindfulness meditation. The result is a highly accessible guide for those interested in healing and wellness. Read the book, put his suggestions to the test in your own life and share the beauty with others."

—FRANK OSTASESKI, FOUNDING DIRECTOR, ZEN HOSPICE PROJECT AND METTA INSTITUTE; NATIONALLY RECOGNIZED EDUCATOR AND COUNSELOR ON SPIRITUALITY IN DYING AND END-OF-LIFE CARE, WHOSE WORK HAS BEEN HONORED BY THE DALAI LAMA AND FEATURED ON BILL MOYER'S TELEVISION SERIES ON OUR OWN TERMS, THE OPRAH WINFREY SHOW, AND IN NUMEROUS PRINT PUBLICATIONS

The Healing Power of Meditation

Your Prescription for Getting Well and Staying Well with Meditation

Gabriel S. Weiss, MD

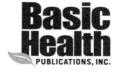
Basic
Health
PUBLICATIONS, INC.

The information contained in this book is based upon the research and personal and professional experiences of the author. It is not intended as a substitute for consulting with your physician or other healthcare provider. Any attempt to diagnose and treat an illness should be done under the direction of a healthcare professional.

The publisher does not advocate the use of any particular healthcare protocol but believes the information in this book should be available to the public. The publisher and author are not responsible for any adverse effects or consequences resulting from the use of the suggestions, preparations, or procedures discussed in this book. Should the reader have any questions concerning the appropriateness of any procedures or preparation mentioned, the author and the publisher strongly suggest consulting a professional healthcare advisor.

Basic Health Publications, Inc.
28812 Top of the World Drive • Laguna Beach, CA 92651
949-715-7327 • www.basichealthpub.com

Publishing credits—Excerpts from *The Feeling of What Happens: Body and Emotion in the Making of Consciousness,* copyright © 1999 by Antonio Damasio, reprinted by permission of Harcourt, Inc.; from *Looking for Spinoza: Joy, Sorrow, and the Feeling Brain,* copyright © 2003 by Antonio Damasio, reprinted by permission of Harcourt, Inc.; from *Full Catastrophe Living* by Jon Kabat-Zinn, copyright © 1990 by Jon Kabat-Zinn, used by permission of Dell Publishing, a division of Random House, Inc.; "Seeing Emotions Through the Eyes of Impermanence," from *No Death, No Fear* by Thich Nhat Hanh, copyright © 2002 by the United Buddhist Church, used by permission of Riverhead Books, an imprint of Penguin Group (USA) Inc.; from *This Is Your Brain on Music* by David J. Levitin, copyright © 2006 by David J. Levitin, used by permission of Dutton, a division of Penguin Group (USA) Inc.; from *Wider Than the Sky* by Gerald M. Edelman, copyright © 2004 by Gerald M. Edelman, reprinted by permission of Yale University Press.

Library of Congress Cataloging-in-Publication Data

Weiss, Gabriel S.
    The healing power of meditation / by Gabriel S. Weiss.
        p. cm.
    Includes bibliographical references and index.
    ISBN 978-1-59120-246-2
    1. Meditation—Health aspects. 2. Meditation—Therapeutic use. I. Title.
    RC489.M43W45   2008
    615.8'51—dc22
                                                                    2008031210

Editor: Cheryl Hirsch
Typesetting/Book design: Gary A. Rosenberg
Cover design: Mike Stromberg

Printed in the United States of America

10 9 8 7 6 5 4 3 2 1

Contents

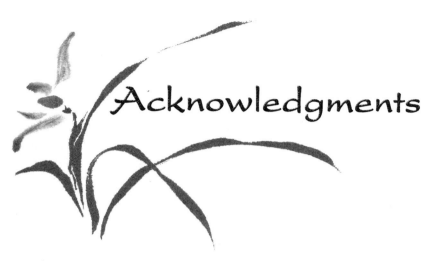

Acknowledgments

Jackie Benington Weiss is my partner on what we call "the long strange trip." She has fearlessly come with me on this journey into exploring meditation and Zen. She is usually my first confidante to read and help edit my writings and offers me much-needed encouragement.

Greg O'Leary is my boyhood friend with a great, wry sense of humor. He is an accomplished attorney and a former graduate literature student at Stanford University, who has remained a lifelong soul mate. He is someone with whom I can talk for hours on end, and never get bored, or run out of things to say. After reading early drafts of this book, he gave me suggestions that led to me further embellishing and "fleshing out" some previously sketchy ideas.

I thank my perceptive and knowledgeable literary agent Bill Gladstone of Waterside Productions, Inc. Bill immediately saw that a book written by a practicing internal medicine doctor, who linked specific meditation exercises to specific illnesses, was something new and different. He helped orient me to the publishing business, and quickly found an excellent publisher for my book.

Norman Goldfind is president and founder of Basic Health Publications, Inc. He founded his publishing company with a mission of helping people make choices that would lead them to optimum health and enhance the quality of their lives. Norm is a wonderfully simpatico person, who supported me in bringing my book to fruition in the form that I wanted, including encouraging me to record the *Teaching Meditation* audio CD that accompanies this book.

I am very grateful to my excellent editor, Cheryl Hirsch. Cheryl's thorough and astute critique of the manuscript, as well as her literary professionalism, organizational abilities, clarity of thought, and her many insights greatly helped to unify the substance and style of this book.

Gary Rosenberg's book design and typesetting skills deserve special recognition. Gary's design artistry and his deep knowledge of publishing industry computer software have combined to produce an attractive, uncrowded book design, which enhances the spiritual feeling of the book and is easy to read. Mike Stromberg's beautiful cover design is also very much appreciated.

The creative talents of Zen artist Rosemary KimBal, the illustrator, are a great fit for this book. See her biography in the section "About the Illustrator." Rosemary's "dancing brush" and her lovely black ink paintings capture the free spirit of meditation.

Much appreciation goes to my spiritual ancestors, including fine authors like Ram Dass, Paramahansa Yogananda, Alan Watts, and Jon Kabat-Zinn, who sparked my interest in meditation and Eastern philosophy. However, my most important spiritual influence is the venerable Thich Nhat Hanh—Zen master, teacher, poet, author, philosopher, and *sangha* (community) builder. Reading his numerous books, sitting in the Ocean of Peace Meditation Hall at Deer Park Monastery while listening to many of his *Dharma* talks, and walking in his footsteps as he led the sangha in walking meditation along the beautiful paths of Deer Park has been for me a constant source of inspiration. Observing, talking to, and practicing with the monks and nuns at Deer Park Monastery has shown me that the beautiful teachings of Buddha can actually work in reality to create a community of harmony.

I also have to acknowledge my medical ancestors, particularly the superb medical scientists and clinicians who mentored me at Stanford University Medical School. Another medical influence on me was the brilliant medical diagnostician and patient-centered humanitarian Sir William Osler (1849–1919), whose life story inspired me to choose internal medicine. It was Dr. Osler who famously said, "Listen to the patient, he's telling you the diagnosis."

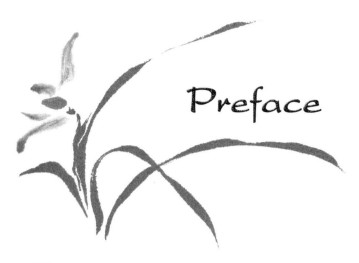

Preface

Discovering the healing power of meditation began for me as a long journey many years ago. And, in the words of the Grateful Dead in their famous song "Truckin'," "What a long strange trip it's been." In 1966, near the sun-drenched, surfing beaches of La Jolla, I entered college at the brand new University of California at San Diego (UCSD) and initially planned to major in physics or chemistry. I later settled on biology as my major (with a minor in philosophy), and studied the rapidly developing new field of microbiology as taught by the pioneering "young lions" of the UCSD biology faculty.

Starting the summer before my freshman year, I had the good fortune to receive a student work-study grant to work in the lab of a man who was, for years, my mentor. Professor Kent R. Wilson, PhD, of the UCSD Chemistry Department was a very creative scientist who was also interested in the arts. Kent had red cheeks, twinkling eyes, and a long, flowing, reddish brown beard. His research used lasers and molecular beams to study the molecular dynamics of what happens to atoms over time as chemical reactions take place. We also produced several computer-animated movies to portray this data, which I wrote and directed.

During my junior year, at another lab at nearby Scripps Institute of Oceanography, I assisted with neurobiology research studying the activation of neurons that transmit information from the eye of the horseshoe crab to its brain. At that time, I concluded it would be unlikely that science would, during my working lifetime, understand the orders-of-magnitude more complex biology of how thinking takes place and how the mind works in general. But I have later found that contemporary neurobiology research is starting to prove me wrong, and there are many exciting developments in this field.

I first became interested in meditation and Eastern spiritual ideas as an undergraduate after reading two amazing books: *Be Here Now* by Ram Dass and *Autobiography of a Yogi* by Paramahansa Yogananda. But the references in those books to multiple gods and goddesses struck me as an unsatisfying explanation of how nature really works. Nevertheless, I found that Yogananda's Self-Realization Fellowship Ashram Center, in nearby Encinitas, California, was a beautiful place to meditate while sitting on the high cliffs overlooking the Pacific Ocean at Swami's Beach.

In 1970, after starting medical school at Stanford University, I took several formal classes in Transcendental Meditation (TM). I practiced meditation sporadically while in medical school. I would often meditate to reduce stress or to boost my energy when running on too little sleep (a frequent problem for medical students). I also noticed that meditation often increased imagination and creativity. During and right after meditation, creative ideas would often spontaneously "bubble up" to the surface of my awareness.

During my internal medicine residency at the University of Oregon in Portland, I became interested in whole-person (holistic) health care, and how alternative and complementary techniques such as meditation, massage, and music therapy could be used to heal symptoms of stress. That approach to treating stress seemed preferable to prescribing tranquilizers that often cause adverse side effects.

For thirty years now I have had a successful, satisfying, and interesting career as a primary-care internal-medicine physician, first in Oregon, later at Scripps Clinic in San Diego County, and now in private practice with two medical offices in Oceanside and San Marcos, California.

As part of my medical practice, I founded the Asclepius Wellness Center in Oceanside, where for years I have taught meditation and music therapy (combining healing with another lifelong passion of mine for playing trumpet). The Asclepius Wellness Center has also developed an integrative referral network to other complementary healthcare providers of chiropractic, acupuncture, and massage therapy, as well as to dietitians and exercise fitness trainers. Over the years, I have been surprised by how few of my medical colleagues pay attention to these non-medication methods of healing.

For a long while, it had seemed to me that it should be possible to extend the quality of the meditative state beyond the time that one is formally meditating. The desire to extend the benefits of meditation into the rest of the activities of my daily life led me to the study of Zen Buddhism and the practice of mindfulness.

The proximity of Deer Park Monastery in nearby Escondido, California, provided me an opportunity to attend many *Dharma* (Zen teachings) talks by Zen master Thich Nhat Hanh and practice walking meditation with the Deer Park community on the monastery grounds. It was at Deer Park that Thich Nhat Hanh gave me what is called my dharma name (community name), which is Compassionate Service of the Heart.

Eventually, I could easily see the compatibility between Western scientific explanations about the forces of nature and the Zen Buddhist description about the nature of reality. This insight has helped inform me about how to seek a path with heart in these two seemingly incongruent worlds, and how meditation and the healing arts are complementary practices.

Come with me on a journey through the pages, ideas, and meditation exercises in this book. It will be good for your health, and may even enhance your joy and passion for the wonders of life.

Introduction

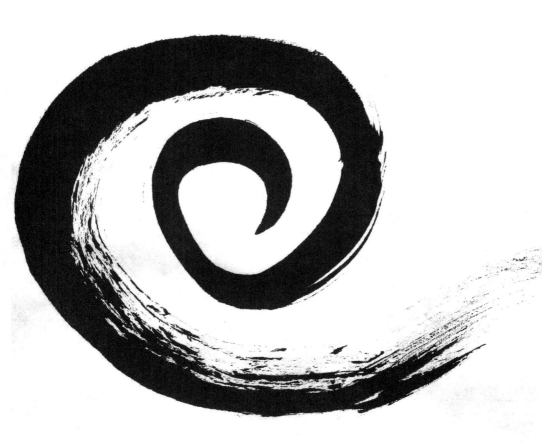

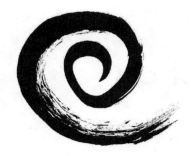 You have an amazing capacity for self-healing. This book explains how to unlock that self-healing power by practicing meditation for a few minutes a day. This simple but deep practice can be used, for example, to reduce the adverse health consequences of stress, to treat chronic pain syndromes, or to diminish the need for medication to treat high blood pressure.

Since I began my career as a primary care internist thirty years ago, I have been providing general medical care for adults, both in my outpatient offices and in the hospital. This long experience has taught me a lot about illness, healing, and wellness. Over the years, the teaching of meditation has become an important part of my practice of medicine. This book describes how meditation can be a powerful tool for healing a whole host of medical conditions. The list of conditions that can be helped by the practice of meditation is quite long. It includes common and serious health problems like heart disease, high blood pressure, cancer, stomach ulcers, asthma, influenza, irritable bowel syndrome (IBS), headache, chronic pain, fibromyalgia, insomnia, obesity, menopausal symptoms, premenstrual syndrome (PMS), psoriasis, chronic fatigue, stress, anxiety, depression, and recovery from surgery.

The Healing Power of Meditation teaches you how to meditate, and explains how the practice of meditation can help to heal health problems, increase your happiness, and reduce human suffering. A biological explanation for the healing power of meditation is revealed.

The material presented here derives from wisdom gained from helping numerous patients recover from illness, as well as from lecture notes developed over my years of teaching meditation classes to patients, nurses, doctors, hospice counselors, and others. The perspective of this book is different from most books about meditation in that it is written by a doctor whose career and passion has been devoted to serving people as they cope with ill health in all of its many manifestations. Presented here are specific diseases and conditions that are linked to specific salutary meditation exercises. Also, since most people have limited time for formal daily meditation exercises, this book explains how to carry over the meditation practice into the whole day by using an approach that is called "the practice of mindfulness."

There are many people who have previously learned a meditation technique, but who don't practice it regularly. And they forget to make the time for meditation when they need it the most, such as when they are under extreme stress. This is because these people haven't learned how to integrate the practice of meditation into the other activities of their daily life. But, in order to benefit the most from meditation, it should be practiced on a regular basis. This is why it is important to develop a philosophy of life that links the practice of meditation to a compatible worldview. I call the worldview presented in this book the "Zen perspective." When people can connect their philosophy of life to the practice of meditation, it deepens their motivation to practice regularly. Then, when they personally feel the healing power of meditation, it becomes even more self-reinforcing.

In addition to teaching patients about meditation, the Zen perspective has been integrated into my medical practice in other ways. This perspective contains a set of concepts that can help people cope with the suffering of illness *whether or not they know how to meditate.* Discussing Zen concepts of impermanence, interconnectedness, compassion, relief of suffering, nonattachment, and happiness become ways of teaching patients how to cope with serious healthcare problems. This is whole-person health care—healing that involves the body, mind, and spirit.

Jacob Bronowski, PhD, the well-known British mathematician, scientist, and humanitarian, insisted that all science is philosophy. He called it "natural philosophy." In *The Ascent of Man* (Little, Brown, 1973) he wrote, "My ambition here has been to create a philosophy that is all of one piece . . . For me the understanding of nature has as its goal the understanding of human nature, and of the human condition within nature." *The Healing Power of Meditation* attempts to connect meditation and its healing power to a "natural philosophy," a Zen-like perspective that accurately reflects the human condition within nature. It is the fruit of combining Eastern meditation practices with a Western scientific understanding of nature.

The book is divided into seven chapters. Following is a brief overview of what you can expect to learn in each chapter.

- **Chapter 1**, Meditation and Wellness, defines what meditation is, and describes the benefits that can come from practicing it. Most importantly, using detailed step-by-step practice instructions, this section teaches you how to meditate. The practice of mindfulness is explained.

- **Chapter 2**, Healing Illness, presents medical case histories, anecdotes, and advice about how meditation can be used to help heal many common illnesses and maladies. Relevant medical research studies are reviewed. Whole-person health care is outlined.

- **Chapter 3**, Zen Perspective, describes how to reduce suffering and enhance well-being by practicing a balanced life of wisdom, morality, and meditation. This chapter also illustrates the healing synergism that occurs when we apply the practice of meditation within the context of a Zen-like philosophy of life. More details about the practice of mindfulness are reviewed. A perspective on birth and death is offered. Read a brief history of the origin of Zen.

- **Chapter 4**, Meditation and Healing Exercises for Expanding Your Practice, presents a series of traditional practices and contemporary meditations to help you reinforce the key Zen concepts presented in Chapter 3 and expand the benefits of formal meditation practice into the whole day. Included are descriptions of how to practice walking meditation, special breathing exercises, music meditation, an exercise called Meditation on the Whole Person, and other alternate meditation exercises. This chapter also explains how to use meditation techniques to reduce physical pain and transform anger.

- **Chapter 5**, Advanced Meditation Concepts for Deepening Your Practice, provides details on how the practice of meditation can be routinely applied throughout the day to reduce anxiety, fear, frustration, and other negative states of mind that interfere with well-being. Ways to promote positive states of mind like joy and compassion, as well as ways to encourage insight are described. This chapter also illustrates how to remain mindful while doing some common daily activities such as being at work or driving the car. Explore Zen concepts about the "self," the community (*sangha*), true love, and the "ultimate dimension."

- **Chapter 6**, Mindful Art, demonstrates that the arts give us one of the most direct ways we have to express the feeling and practice of meditation and Zen. This chapter contains excerpts from mindful poems, songs, and literature, plus examples of meditative painting, calligraphy, sculpture art, and photography.

- **Chapter 7**, The Nature of Reality and Consciousness, compares a Western scientific understanding about the nature of reality and how the mind works to key aspects of meditation and Zen teachings. Evolution, feelings, consciousness, learning, and wisdom are some of the topics explored. The chapter ends with an explanation of the neurobiology of how meditation works to heal the mind and body. This summation provides a scientific understanding of what is going on inside the brain during meditation and the mechanisms that give meditation its power to heal.

This book is probably best read a few pages at a time to let the information sink in slowly. I encourage you to try the meditation exercises before proceeding to the next chapter. Resist the urge to rush through the chapters. Putting the ideas and exercises into practice as you read will be more beneficial to you and your health.

CHAPTER ONE

Meditation and Wellness

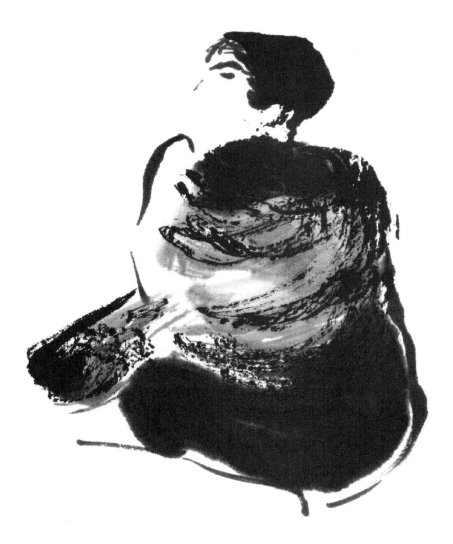

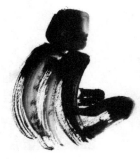

Meditation is a healing practice. As a doctor, I have incorporated meditation into my medical practice. Over the years, I have seen many patients benefit from the healing power of meditation. I often encounter patients with problems that won't respond to medication, but will resolve or lessen with meditation. Compared to medication treatment, healing using meditation also has the great advantage of having no risk of adverse side effects, and it's free!

I have witnessed the practice of meditation help a retired engineer overcome a serious depression. An anxious widow, whose blood pressure could not be controlled with medication alone, learned to avoid severe blood pressure spikes by practicing meditation. A man with advanced-stage lung cancer, by meditating, found the peace and inner strength that enabled him to undergo chemotherapy with a positive attitude. An elderly woman, who had long suffered in an abusive marriage, through meditation, was finally able to find the self-esteem to live on her own and is now much happier pursuing many other interests. A young healthcare worker, who frequently missed work days due to psychosomatic, stress-induced symptoms, found in meditation a way to bring her life back into a healthy balance. Meditation has also helped people suffering from chronic insomnia learn to return to sleep naturally.

In addition to practicing sitting meditation, I practice walking meditation (a form of movement meditation) every day when I walk from my office in Oceanside, California, to nearby Tri-City Medical Center, where I hospitalize my sickest patients. This allows me to arrive at my patients' bedside in a clear-minded, creative, and compassionate state of mind to help guide their hospital care.

This book reveals the surprising power of meditation to heal our mind and body. This self-healing aspect of meditation has been known for thousands of years. But we are only recently coming to find the scientific basis for why it has this capacity. This is not a book about religion. The Zen perspective presented here is compatible with all major world religions. And, as you shall see, this perspective is also consistent with the current scientific understanding of the laws of nature and how the mind works.

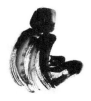

SKILLFUL MEANS

Have you ever wondered how the pieces of your life fit together? What purpose do they serve? There are so many pieces of your life to consider: food, sleep, work, exercise, spending time with family and friends, household duties, raising kids, caring for aging parents, helping other people, walking the dog, listening to music, other recreational activities, reading, thinking, planning, and on and on. How much time should you devote to each of these activities? What is their relative importance? Should you spend less time with one activity so you have more time for others?

Rather than consider each of these aspects individually, it is helpful to look at your life as a process that unfolds on two levels. The first level is biological: the underlying physical nature of your existence and the laws that govern the universe. This is the physical dimension of your life. The second level is your worldview: the psychological and philosophical way you view the world, which motivates much of your actions. This is the spiritual dimension of your life.

It is possible to use skillful means to forge a harmonious connection between the physical and spiritual aspects of our lives. The practice of meditation is the skillful means we can use to forge that link and bring our lives into a balance. This practice enhances our happiness, reduces suffering, helps heal illness, and promotes physical well-being.

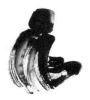

WHAT IS MEDITATION?

Meditation is a state of awareness of the present without thinking. In our normal state of consciousness, the thinking mind is usually replaying or regretting the past, or planning or worrying about the future. However, meditation is about keeping our awareness totally focused on what is happening in the present moment. This allows us to be in touch with the wonders of the present, without any discursive, verbal thinking getting in the way.

In order to meditate, we must quiet the interminable chatter that goes on inside our heads. Then, when the thinking mind goes silent, this allows us to reach a *different state of consciousness,* a here-and-now, pres-ent-oriented awareness called meditation. In this state, we are no longer doing or thinking; we are simply being. Techniques you will learn and practice will enable you to easily enter this meditative state. But first, let's examine some of the evidence for the healing power of meditation.

PHYSICAL HEALTH EFFECTS

Meditation is more than a psychological phenomenon. Medical research shows that meditation is associated with many reproducible physical changes in the brain and the body. Consider a few of these scientific findings.

Herbert Benson, a cardiologist and pioneer in mind-body medicine, was the first to conduct medical research on meditation in the United States. In the early 1970s at Boston's Beth Israel Hospital and Harvard Medical School, Dr. Benson studied meditators who used a mantra-based meditation technique called Transcendental Meditation and found that the meditation lowered blood pressure, heart rate, breathing, and metab-olism. Dr. Benson called this phenomenon the "relaxation response," and in his classic book, *The Relaxation Response* (HarperCollins, 1975), he characterized it as an "inducible physiologic state of quietude." The phys-ical changes that result from meditation seemed to Dr. Benson to be the opposite of a well-known set of physiologic responses to stressful situa-tions that humans have inherited through evolution called the "fight-or-flight response." About the relaxation response phenomenon, Dr. Benson further observed, "Indeed, our progenitors handed down to us a second, equally essential survival mechanism—the ability to heal and rejuvenate our bodies."

In addition to the potentially beneficial cardiovascular effects of lower blood pressure and heart rate, newer medical research has looked at other possible health benefits of meditation. One study of immune function found that meditators, when given flu shot, have a much larg-er antibody response (produce more influenza-fighting antibodies). In another study of immune function, breast cancer patients who medi-tate, compared to others who didn't, were found to have increased num-bers of natural killer white blood cells. These are the most efficient white blood cells at seeking out and killing cancer cells and fighting off virus infections.

Another clinical study conducted by Blue Shield insurance company found that surgery patients who listened to a guided meditation (a form of meditation that uses phrases or evocative spoken images to guide the mind into a relaxed meditative state) audio CD before surgery recovered from surgery more quickly, cost an average of two thousand dollars less per surgery, and reported a greater sense of healing.

At the University of Massachusetts Stress Reduction Clinic, one of the most respected stress and pain clinics in the country, meditation has been shown to reduce chronic pain by an average of 50 percent. Follow-up studies showed the pain reduction lasted for more than a year.

Research studies using electroencephalograms (EEGs) performed on people while they were meditating found that brain waves in various parts of their brain became more harmonically in sync. EEGs performed during meditation reveal a shift away from alpha waves that are associated with conscious thought, toward more predominance of theta waves that dominate the brain during periods of deep relaxation.

In recent years, medical science has developed powerful new tools to scan the living brain to look for localized differences in metabolism and blood flow in various regions. Imaging scans done on people while meditating have shown objective evidence of physiologic changes occurring within the brain during meditation. For example, functional magnetic resonance imaging (fMRI) and positron emission tomography (PET) brain scans have found that there are regional changes in blood flow and metabolism that occur in various parts of the brain during meditation.

Some parts of the brain become more metabolically active during meditation, such as the left prefrontal cortex (a region associated with happiness and positive thoughts) and the limbic system (the part of the brain that generates emotional responses) deep in the subcortex of the brain. Some regions of the brain become very inactive, such as other parts of the frontal lobe (where reasoning and planning take place), and parts of the parietal lobe (which handles muscle and sensory functions). Richard Davidson, a neuroscientist at the University of Wisconsin, studied Buddhist monks during meditation. He found that during meditation the areas of the brain that are normally associated with happiness and empathy "light up" on an MRI brain scan.

These are only a few examples. We will be going into more depth about the research and physical benefits of meditation in Chapter 2.

PSYCHOLOGICAL BENEFITS

The subjective evidence of the psychological effects of meditation, as reported by countless meditators over the centuries, is also important. People who meditate consistently report that meditation results in an increased feeling of happiness, freshness, peace, and freedom. On the audiobook *Alan Watts Teaches Meditation* (Audio Renaissance, 1992), Watts says, "Meditation is a kind of digging the present. It's a kind of grooving with the Eternal Now. It brings us into a state of peace where we can understand that point of life, the place where it's at, is simply here and now."

Meditating increases happiness by promoting positive states of mind such as compassion, kindness, love, generosity, patience, and tolerance. The calm and insights that occur as a result of meditation (see next section) can also help heal symptoms of severe stress, feelings of loss, loneliness, pain, frustration, anger, despair, and even fear of impending death. As will be explained further in Chapter 2, the positive states of mind created by meditation are an integral part of the physical healing process.

THE BENEFIT OF INSIGHT

Herbert Benson came to understand what he called the "two-step process" described by advanced practitioners of meditation, like Tibetan monks. According to Dr. Benson in his foreword to *The Relaxation Response:* "First, you evoke the relaxation response [or a meditative state] and reap its healthful reward. Then, when your mind is quiet, when focusing has opened a door in your mind, visualize an outcome that is meaningful for you."

Another way of describing this two-step process is that, once you create a calm center and enter the nonthinking state of "alert stillness" called meditation, insights may "bubble up" to the surface of your awareness.

Not as the end result of a reasoning, thinking process, but more like a sudden creative inspiration. These insights help you look deeply into the root causes of your physical and mental problems, and help you see clearly how to reduce your suffering, and the suffering of others.

The process of attaining these insights is made easier if one has previously developed an understanding of impermanence, interconnectedness, nonattachment, and compassion. These concepts and their integration into your life will be discussed in great detail in later chapters. I will first describe how to meditate.

Read the next section when you are able to practice the meditation exercises at the same time.

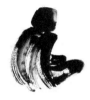

LEARNING TO MEDITATE

There is no one best way to meditate. If you haven't previously learned how to meditate, the instructions below will give you a good start. If you already practice meditation and have a meditation method you like, you should continue to practice that method. For advanced meditators, the following meditation exercises, the exercises described later in the book, and the *Teaching Meditation* audio CD that accompanies this book can all provide possible alternate ways to expand your meditation practice. The other material in this book can deepen your practice by showing you the many positive effects meditation can have on health and healing.

FOCUS ON A MANTRA

To make it easier to enter the meditative state and to help free the mind from discursive verbal thinking, it can be extremely useful to focus the mind instead on a sound. As when a bell or gong sounds, this type of pure sound cuts through the world of symbols and just "is." No thinking is necessary to appreciate the sound. And, while you are focused on the sound, the thinking process is temporarily suppressed. But, whereas the sound of a bell quickly fades, a chanted mantra is a sound that can be sustained as a focus for meditation for a much longer time.

The word "mantra" is Sanskrit for "that which frees the mind." A mantra is a chanted word or sound that is used, not for its meaning, but for the quality of the sound it makes. A mantra can be chanted out loud or repeated internally and silently in your "mind's ear." One of the most common mantras, used for more than two thousand years, is the sound "OM" or "AUM." Don Campbell, a leading music therapist, says in his book *The Mozart Effect* (Harper, 2001) that "OM" and "AHH" are two of the most powerful sounds for evoking the relaxation response. Later in this chapter you will learn to use both of these sounds in one mantra.

But first, practice saying "OM" out loud. Try chanting that sound for several minutes right now.

1. Sit upright and chant "OOOOOOMMMMM" slowly for a few minutes, over and over again, in a deep voice. Use any volume, from softly humming to a loud, resonant sound. Close your eyes and take a slow, deep in-breath. Then, as you release your out-breath, let the sound of "OOOOOOMMMMM" flow out easily and freely, like you might imagine monks and nuns slowly chanting in unison. Feel a sense of relaxation and release, or "letting go," as you say "OM."

2. Next, practice chanting "OM" silently, which is like hearing "OM" repeated in your "mind's ear." Close your eyes and take a slow, deep in-breath. Then, as you release your out-breath, listen to the sound of "OOOOOOMMMMM" in your mind's ear. Try that for a couple of minutes. If you have trouble staying concentrated on hearing the sound internally, let yourself hum it softly out loud again. Notice the "feel" of the sound of "OM" resonating in your sinus cavities. Then chant "OM" ever more softly until it can only be felt and heard silently.

FOCUS ON THE BREATH

A second technique to help you enter the meditative state is to focus awareness on the breath. If you use a silent mantra as the focus for meditation, most of "the action" takes place in your head. But, focusing awareness on your breath links your mind to your body. Try meditating by focusing on breath for a few minutes right now.

1. Remain still and upright, close your eyes and take a slow, deep in-breath, and then release your out-breath. Notice everything about your breath, being especially aware of breathing in and breathing out. Focus on the feeling of the flow of air entering your nostrils and filling up your lungs. Or you might choose to focus on the outward and inward breathing movements of your abdomen, diaphragm, and chest. Or you can pay attention to the sensations of a small area below the nose and above the upper lip as air flows in and out of the nostrils. (If possible, it is preferable to breathe in through the nose in order to humidify and filter the air, and to avoid getting a dry mouth.) Meditate on your breath like this for several minutes.

Another useful meditation technique is to feel the effect of breathing heavily. This hyperventilation "trick" can transiently stop your thinking mind and briefly simulate the feeling of a deep meditative state.

1. While sitting, take eight or ten rapid, deep breaths, in and out, followed by a slow exhalation through pursed lips. You may at first feel some brief lightheadedness. Then after that, notice the pleasant feeling of a nonthinking, settled awareness that occurs. This peaceful feeling will fade away after a couple of minutes, whereas meditation can sustain that state for a much longer period of time. However, this heavy-breathing exercise will give the novice meditator some idea of the feeling of deeper meditation, which can help one learn, by feel, how to more quickly enter into a deep meditative state.

LET THOUGHTS FADE AWAY

During meditation, thinking inevitably reasserts itself. When you notice this, don't get angry and try to force the thoughts out—that would disrupt the quiet stillness you are trying to develop in your mind. It would be like trying to smooth rough water with a big broom; it would only disturb it all the more. Simply bring your awareness gently back to your breath or mantra. Allow the thoughts to simply fade away like other background sounds—like waves crashing on the beach or wind blowing through leaves in the trees.

ESTABLISHING A DAILY MEDITATION: AH-OM BREATH

Now we get to the meditation method I would like you to try practicing regularly. I call this method AH-OM Breath meditation. It links awareness of your breath to awareness of the sound of a mantra. I like the combination of focusing on both *breath* and *sound* because it is more mentally absorbing than either alone—and thus makes it easier to stay concentrated in meditation. (When I use either only sound, or only breath, as the sole focus for meditation, I find my mind wandering off into thinking more of the time.)

During AH-OM Breath meditation, stay concentrated the entire time on the sensations associated with breathing. And, at the same time, also focus on a mantra sound. The sound you will focus on is a silently chanted, two-syllable mantra: "AH-OM."

"AH," the first syllable of the mantra, is pronounced like the first syllable in the word "amen." "AH" also sounds like the sound of inhaling. You are already familiar with the sound of "OM."

To practice AH-OM Breath meditation, it is necessary to combine hearing the sound of "AH" and "OM" together with maintaining a focused awareness on your breath, as explained in more detail below. Read the instructions through first.

1. Sit in a comfortable chair or, if you prefer, on a cushion on the floor. Sit in an upright, centered posture so your breath can flow freely. If sitting in a chair, keep your legs uncrossed with your feet flat on the floor. Consciously relax the muscles in your face, jaw, shoulders, and arms. It is okay to keep your eyes closed, half-open, or open. A light, Buddha-like smile helps.

2. When you inhale, silently say or hear "AAAAHHHHH." And, at the same time, concentrate your awareness on your entire in-breath *all the way through* to the end of the in-breath.

3. When you exhale (longer than inhalation) hear "OOOOOMMMM" in your "mind's ear," while focusing attention on your entire out-breath. Stay concentrated on your breath, moment to moment, *all the way through* to the end of the out-breath.

Meditate using the above AH-OM Breath technique for fifteen to thirty minutes once or twice a day as a regular practice. Time it with a watch. Find a quiet place where you won't be interrupted. I usually like to meditate first thing in the morning before the rest of the day starts. Sometimes I may do it on a lunch break in my car. But any time is okay.

Remember, when thoughts occur to let them simply fade away. While meditation is relaxing and stress relieving, you don't just allow yourself to dissipate. Meditation requires concentration. The more you practice, the better you learn how to concentrate and focus your awareness.

Try practicing AH-OM Breath meditation right now.

MANY PATHS TO MEDITATION

The method of meditating just described is not the only good way to meditate. AH-OM Breath meditation is not even the only way that I meditate. It is, however, the meditation method I use most frequently as the foundation for my daily practice. It is composed of age-old elements that are easily learned and work very well.

Transcendental Meditation, breath meditation in the Zen or Yoga tradition, guided meditation, mindfulness meditation, walking meditation, t'ai chi, qi gong, Relaxation Response meditation, Mindfulness-Based Stress Reduction, progressive muscle relaxation exercises, and Vipassana (also called Insight) Meditation are examples of some other good techniques. You can peruse the bibliography at the end of this book for references to other perfectly valid meditation methods. The list contains many books by meditation masters. Reading some of these sources of wisdom can deepen your understanding and practice.

MINDFULNESS, CONCENTRATION, AND INSIGHT

Mindfulness, concentration, and insight are three important elements involved in the deeper practice of meditation—so much so that the Sanskrit words for mindfulness, concentration, and insight, which are *smrti, samadhi,* and *prajna,* are emblazoned on a large stained glass window at the front of the Ocean of Peace Meditation Hall at Deer Park Monastery in Escondido, California (see Plate 1, page 181). This symbolizes that mindfulness applied with concentration produces insight.

Mindfulness represents a process by which you engage in the act of meditating while you are also engaged in performing many of your normal daily activities. So, this expands greatly your opportunity to be meditating far beyond the fifteen to sixty minutes a day a person might spend in formal sitting meditation.

Concentration is the ability to keep your attention on the focus of your meditation, without continually drifting off into thinking. Developing your capacity to concentrate during meditation deepens the stillness of the mind necessary to produce insight.

Gaining insight means to gain the wisdom to understand the root causes of your problems and how to overcome those problems, thereby easing suffering and enhancing your happiness. This is one of the greatest so-called fruits of meditation.

MINDFULNESS

Mindfulness is a form of meditation practiced during normal daily activities. But, when we say mindfulness, what is your mind full of? Certainly not thoughts, since meditation is not about thinking. Instead, mindfulness is keeping your mind full of what's happening in the present moment. It is a way of paying attention and staying totally focused on what you are doing *right now*—with no discursive thinking or talking getting in the way of the immediacy of the experience.

The opposite of mindfulness is forgetfulness, which is what happens when you dwell in the past or worry about the future; you don't notice what's going on in the present so you lose touch with yourself. You try to do, or pay attention to, too many things at once and, as a result, focus on none of them adequately. You forget where you put an object you were just holding in your hand. In the end, this scatter-minded and forgetful state produces frustration and saps energy and purpose.

The title of a book by Jon Kabat-Zinn captures the concept of mindfulness this way: *Wherever You Go, There You Are* (Hyperion, 1994). Kabat-Zinn is founder and director of the University of Massachusetts

Stress Reduction Clinic, which has pioneered methods for reducing chronic pain through meditation. He writes that, when we lose touch with where we are and what we are doing right now,

> We fall into a robot-like way of seeing and thinking and doing. In those moments, we break contact with what is deepest in ourselves and affords us perhaps our greatest opportunities for creativity, learning, and growing. If we are not careful, these clouded moments can stretch out and become most of our lives. To allow ourselves to be truly in touch with where we already are, no matter where that is, we have to pause in our experience long enough to let the present moment sink in; long enough to actually *feel* the present moment, to see it in its fullness, to hold it in awareness and thereby come to know and understand it better.

Mindfulness, or awareness of what is happening in the present moment, should be practiced not just during sitting meditation, but also during ordinary daily activities such as walking, eating, bathing, urinating, brushing your teeth, getting dressed in the morning, stretching, breathing, or doing yard work and simple labor. With mindfulness meditation the activity, itself, becomes the focus of your meditation, as you concentrate your attention on the moment-to-moment awareness of what it is you are experiencing or doing right now. A few examples follow: If you are sweeping your porch, the movements of your hands, arms, and the broom can be the focus for your meditation. If you are walking, the movements and sensations in your feet can be the focus. If you are eating, you can pay close attention to your hand picking up a spoon and then bringing the food to your mouth; and then become immersed in all the marvelous smells, tastes, and sensations involved in eating and swallowing each bite. By simply paying attention, in a non-critical way, you quiet thinking and keep yourself grounded in a present awareness.

Formal sitting meditation, which is also a form of mindfulness, gives you an opportunity to stop all of your "doing" and *practice* being fully concentrated in the present moment for a brief fifteen to thirty minutes. Practicing mindfulness during other daily activities allows you to apply that meditative state of consciousness to the larger period in your life when you are not engaged in formal sitting meditation practice. So, in a sense, sitting meditation also functions as a type of "rehearsal," helping you to learn how to stay mindfully present during many other activities and doings of your daily life. Practicing sitting meditation helps teach you that, during the rest of your day, you should avoid rushing ahead by staying mindfully in the moment, one step at a time. For more about the practice of mindfulness, see Chapters 3 and 5 on the Zen Perspective and Advanced Meditation Concepts.

CONCENTRATION

Meditation is a practice. One has to practice meditation regularly to develop the concentration necessary to allow one to achieve a deep state of meditation. I know that I am getting into a deep meditative state when it seems like my mind is becoming as calm and still as a reflecting pool of clear water on a windless day, and then maintains that state of alert stillness for an extended period of time. I may often feel a sensation of release of tension, and then a feeling inside of open space and peace. Concentration is also necessary to remain focused in mindfulness for an extended period of time while engaged in normal daily activities.

When you develop an ability to stay concentrated in meditation, you go beyond the world of symbols into the silence of a deep present awareness, an alert stillness. During meditation, as your mind becomes very quiet, the sound of your mantra may eventually fade away into the background, which allows you to be aware of other sounds in the environment. The "tide" of your in-breath and out-breath merges with a larger awareness. There may seem very little separation between yourself and the world of nature outside you. It all becomes "one big happening."

INSIGHT

In meditation, when one remains concentrated in a state of alert stillness, something very special then occurs: stillness speaks (which is the title of one of writer Eckhart Tolle's books, published by New World Library, 2003). When stillness speaks to us, we may then acquire wisdom and become aware of creative and original insights. As described in another Tolle book, *A New Earth* (Dutton, 2005), this shift in consciousness is a type of "awakening." Acquiring this meditative wisdom allows us to awaken to the root causes of life's problems. And we obtain insight about what we need to do to reduce life's suffering and enhance our physical and spiritual well-being.

It is worth emphasizing that it is the regular practice of meditation that helps develop your concentration. Greater concentration allows you to go deeper into meditative silence, which then helps to promote the occurrence of spontaneous insight. So, when you are experiencing stress, illness, or emotional negativity, remember to take the time to practice meditation, which then results in acquiring the wisdom needed to transform and heal your suffering.

PRACTICE REVIEW

The goal of this section is to simply reinforce and review the AH-OM Breath meditation method I began to learn earlier. The repetition of this fundamental technique will form the foundation of our practice of meditation. So let's recall the basic elements of that technique.

1. **Focus on the mantra.** Normally, begin meditation by chanting the AH-OM mantra silently in your "mind's ear." But, to help internalize the sound of "OM," you may want to practice chanting it out loud again for a few minutes right now. Each time you release your breath play with altering the pitch, breathiness, resonance, or humming qualities of the sound of "OM." This keeps the sound interesting and fresh in your mind's ear, helping to keep your awareness concentrated on the sound.

2. **Focus awareness on your breath.** While staying aware of the sound of the internally chanted mantra, also focus awareness on your breath. Notice everything about your breath: especially awareness of breathing in and out through the nose, the feeling of air passing down your throat and into your lungs, and the movements of your abdomen and chest.

3. **Remember to let thoughts fade away.** When thinking inevitably

reasserts itself, do not get angry. Simply bring your awareness gently back to your mantra and breath, and allow the thoughts to simply fade away into the background.

4. **Now combine your awareness of both sound and breath with AH-OM Breath meditation.** When you inhale, silently hear the sound of "AH." And, at the same time, maintain an awareness of your in-breath all the way through. When you exhale—make this longer than the in-hale—internally hear the sound of "OOOOMMMM," and follow your out-breath all the way through. The sounds of "AH" and "OM" may eventually combine to become more like the sound "AHHHH-OOOMMMM," or simply "AUM." Breathing in and out can then become a smooth, continuous motion like the bowing of a violin.

HELPFUL HINTS

- **To stay focused:** If you have trouble staying concentrated on the breath at the same time that you are focusing on the sound of "AH-OM," instead try practicing using the mantra "in-out." The word "in" will remind you to follow your in-breath, and the word "out" will help remind you to stay focused on the entire out-breath. Then, when you feel comfortable that you can maintain this dual focus, try going back to the "AH-OM" mantra.

- **To deal with sleepiness:** The state of consciousness that is meditation is a *waking state* of alert stillness. But you might occasionally find yourself falling asleep during meditation. This means that you are lacking sleep. So just let yourself catch up on the sleep you need.

- **To make meditation a daily experience:** Meditation is a spiritual practice. One has to practice meditation regularly to develop the concentration needed to maintain a sustained state of focused awareness. Practice meditating for fifteen to thirty minutes or more every day. Sit upright, with relaxed forehead and shoulders. A light, Buddha-like smile helps. Remember what to do with thoughts. Try not to try too hard. Just enjoy your breathing.

Practice meditating again right now.

CHAPTER TWO

Healing Illness: A Prescription for Meditation

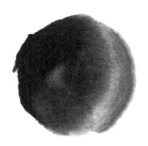

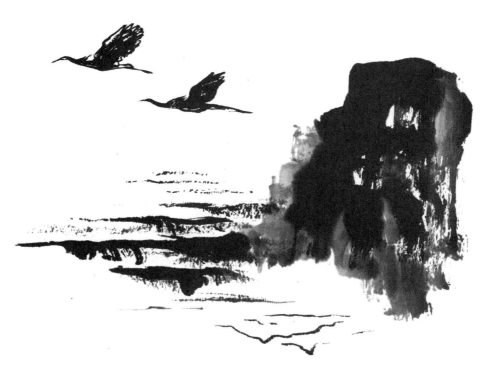

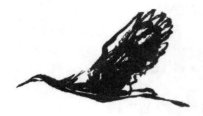

The number of conditions that can be helped by meditation runs the gamut from "A" for asthma to "Z" for can't get enough zzzzz's (insomnia), from cancer and cardiac disease to obesity. This chapter looks in greater detail at the use of meditation in the treatment of illness. If the practice of meditation were routinely applied by patients with one or more of the conditions discussed here, the potential impact on health care and health-care costs would be enormous.

The amount and quality of sound scientific information on the use of meditation to treat illness has grown enormously in recent years. Many of the research studies have demonstrated that treating a variety of medical conditions with meditation is beneficial. It is important to bear in mind though that medical research (or any research for that matter) contains conflicts and contradictions. They are inevitable. And, research studies on meditation are no exception.

Many of the published studies that investigate meditation as a medical treatment are not perfect due to difficulty with designing a meditation experiment. Following are the standard research methods used and the special challenges that the study of meditation poses:

- **Double-blind placebo-controlled study:** In order to avoid observer bias in research, the "gold standard" is to employ what is called a double-blind placebo-controlled study method. But it is difficult to design a study where neither the subject nor the researchers know if the participant is actually meditating!

- **Randomized controlled trial:** The next best type of medical research uses the experimental method called the randomized controlled trial, where study participants with similar characteristics are randomly assigned to different treatment groups. Some of the meditation research studies do not adhere to this standard, but there is an increasing number of randomized controlled trials now published about the use of meditation to alleviate illness. The credibility of these experimental results is greatly enhanced when the positive findings of a randomized clinical trial can be replicated by a similar study performed by an independent investigational group. It is important to note that the experimental results of some of the studies detailed below have yet to be confirmed by a second independent clinical investigation.

Some meditation studies do not include a large enough number of participants to statistically prove that their positive test results are unlikely to be due to chance alone. We are now, however, seeing more meditation studies published along with a statistical analysis that demonstrates their results are statistically significant.

Nevertheless, until more studies come along, we are left with imperfect studies, many of which show a positive benefit from using meditation in the treatment of particular illnesses. Fortunately, meditation practice has not been associated with any harmful side effects, and it's free. So trying it yourself is low risk. You can try it as a mind experiment in the laboratory of your own life and see if it works for you.

However, meditation is not a panacea. It is important to understand that it is only one of many possible treatments. See the section "Whole-Person Health Care" at the end of this chapter for a discussion of health care wherein meditation is only part of the mix of treatment options. Meditation doesn't work for everyone because it takes a commitment of time and energy to practice and apply it. Many people just prefer not to go that route.

The expected time needed to realize benefits from meditation for different medical problems varies depending on the specific condition being treated. If you are treating insomnia that is being caused by not being able to turn off the thinking mind at night, then meditation might start working right away. It will take a much longer meditation practice to transform the fear associated with living with cancer, or to mitigate the pain of chronic arthritis.

The following categories of illness that can be treated with meditation are listed alphabetically. Where possible, specific meditation practices that have been shown to be valuable in treating specific illnesses are identified. The case histories described are real, but the patients' names have been changed for reasons of confidentiality.

CANCER

Meditation can help cancer patients in three ways. First, meditation can reduce fear and depression, as well as restore a sense of calm and peace, in someone who has received the very scary diagnosis of cancer. More will be said about this in the section entitled "Mood and Affective Disorders" later in this chapter. Second, as will be discussed in detail in the section "Meditations for Transforming Pain" in Chapter 4, meditation techniques can reduce cancer pain. Third, meditation can help boost the immune system, which is our most powerful self-healing mechanism for attacking and killing cancer cells.

A study of breast cancer patients by Anthony Bakke and associates from the Oregon Health and Science University in Portland, reported in the *Journal of Psychosomatic Research* (2002), found that guided meditation increased the number of the type of white blood cells that attack growing cancer cells. This experiment studied twenty-five women with early-stage breast cancer. These women practiced at least three times weekly using audiotapes that guided them through an exercise of progressive muscle relaxation. They were also asked to visualize their immune cells attacking their cancer. The article describes progressive muscle relaxation as a meditation-like activity: "The purpose of progressive relaxation is to quiet the thoughts and create an inwardly focused state of awareness." This guided meditation technique is very similar to a component in the meditation method called Buddha's Breathing Exercises. (See page 114 for instructions on how to do this meditative technique, which uses the guidewords "calm/ release" to progressively relax the muscles and calm the mind.)

Dr. Bakke's group measured the number of a specific type of lymphocytic white blood cells called natural killers that are known to have a very powerful capacity to attack and kill cancer cells. There was no control group in this study. What they found was that, after eight weeks of guided meditation practice, the women in the study had a statistically significant increase in the numbers of their natural killer cells of approximately 16 percent. By twenty weeks, however, the increase from baseline had diminished to 5 percent. But, the study also found that psychometric measurements of depression still remained much improved three months after the guided meditation intervention.

A randomized controlled clinical trial led by Cecile Lengacher at the University of South Florida studied the effect of guided meditation in twenty-eight breast cancer patients. They measured the ability of their natural killer cells to attack and kill cancer cells—a process called cytotoxicity. The study was designed to see if there were differences in natural killer cell activity (cytotoxicity) between women randomly assigned to the guided meditation group versus a control group. The women who entered the trial all had early-stage breast cancer and had not yet undergone cancer surgery. Blood tests were obtained at baseline and four weeks after surgery. The type of meditation method used in this study was very similar to the progressive muscle relaxation method used in Bakke's study. The control group received standard cancer care, but no meditation. The blood test results showed that four weeks after breast cancer surgery, the meditation group had a highly significant increase—greater than 75 percent—in the cancer-killing capacity of their natural killer white blood cells compared to the control group!

Linda Carlson's group at the University of Calgary in Canada published the results of a randomized clinical trial with fifty-nine breast and prostate cancer patients trained in mindfulness meditation. Their study used a method modeled after the Mindfulness-Based Stress Reduction program at the University of Massachusetts Stress Reduction Clinic developed by Jon Kabat-Zinn, which is described in more detail later in this chapter in the section "Stress." The intervention took place as a once-a-week, ninety-minute group session. They found the meditation group of breast and prostate cancer patients demonstrated significant improvements in their quality of life, symptoms of stress and anxiety, and quality of sleep.

The Dana-Farber/Harvard Cancer Center in Boston published a comprehensive review of clinical trials of meditation used as treatment in cancer patients that concluded, "Meditation has clinically relevant implications to alleviate psychological and physical suffering of persons living with cancer." The following case history from my medical practice illustrates this quite well.

Ari is a very fastidious, nervous-appearing, thin man in his fifties, who came to see me for a general medical checkup. At our first meeting, Ari confided that a year ago a nodule had been detected on his last chest x-ray. He had been so nervous and upset about what it meant that he reacted by completely forcing it out of his mind. He had not pursued any further evaluation of it for more than a year. Our investigation led to a lung biopsy and lung surgery, which proved that the lung nodule was cancer. And it had already spread to several adjacent lymph nodes. Ari was terrified and paralyzed with fear. He couldn't eat, or sleep, or decide whether to undergo the recommended chemotherapy.

At about this same time, Ari began taking a meditation class, and learned the AH-OM Breath meditation technique (see page 16 for instructions). By practicing meditation on a daily basis, Ari was able to lose his feeling of despair and marshal the inner strength he needed to embark on the chemotherapy. Four years later, he seems to be defying very long odds, as his advanced-stage cancer remains in remission on follow-up PET scans. He has also regained his feeling of happiness at being alive. Ari once again enjoys spending time with his wife doing their normal activities such as going out to local restaurants. He has even traveled to a foreign country, Israel, which he had long wanted to visit. After coming back from Israel, Ari was excited to tell me he had learned a new mantra. It was *"shalom"* with the last syllable pronounced with more emphasis and longer than the first syllable. It is interesting that the sound of the mantra *"shalom"* is very similar to the sound of "AH-OM."

CARDIOVASCULAR DISEASE

The category of cardiovascular disease includes high blood pressure, tachycardia (fast heart rate) and dysrhythmia (irregular heartbeat), congestive heart failure and cardiomyopathy (weak heart muscle), coronary artery disease (diseased blood vessels in the heart), angina (chest pain due to diminished blood flow to the heart muscle), and heart attack.

HYPERTENSION

Blood pressure measurements include two numbers; for example, 120/70. The upper number, called the systolic pressure, is the pressure

in the arteries of the body when the heart i.
number, called the diastolic pressure, is the p
the heart is filling up with blood between heart
medical name for high blood pressure. It is on
conditions treated by primary care physicians.
the "silent killer" because the condition usually p.
until it causes a major complication like a heart atta   ⌐ ⌐pathy,
stroke, or kidney failure.

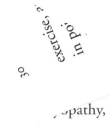

Several clinical trials have shown reductions in blood pressure as a
result of learning a meditation technique. One randomized clinical trial
by Vernon Barnes and colleagues, published in *Psychosomatic Medicine,*
studied the effect of meditation on seventy-three healthy middle-school
adolescents with normal blood pressure. They used a meditation method
that asked the adolescents to focus on the movements of their diaphragm
while breathing in a slow, deep, relaxed manner. The study found that,
compared to the control group, the meditation group had a statistically significant lower blood pressure (5.6 millimeter [mm] lower systolic
and 4.2 mm lower diastolic pressure) and slower heart rate (5.6 beats
per minute slower).

A randomized controlled trial conducted by Maura Paul-Labrador and
associates, published in the *Archives of Internal Medicine* (2006), studied
103 adults with coronary artery heart disease for sixteen weeks. They used
the mantra-based meditation technique called Transcendental Meditation (TM). The group taught TM experienced, on average, a statistically
significant 6.2 mm lower systolic blood pressure than the control group.

Robert Schneider and colleagues published a single-blind randomized
clinical trial of TM in the journal *Hypertension* that studied 213 African
Americans with high blood pressure. The three-month trial compared
TM to a control group treated with a lifestyle modification program.
The group trained in TM experienced a highly significant 10.7 mm drop
in systolic blood pressure and a 6.4 mm drop in diastolic pressure.

However, thus far in the medical literature there have been no published studies that show meditation can sustain long-term reductions in
blood pressure. Therefore, in the treatment of hypertension, meditation
is probably best used to help prevent or treat short-term spikes in blood
pressure elevation, and as a complementary treatment along with diet,

antihypertensive medication. My patient Jeannie is a case
in point.

Jeannie is a sweet woman in her seventies who comes to my office to
have me help manage her hypertension. She is always smiling and very
well dressed with her white hair neatly combed. She lives by herself and
faithfully takes her blood pressure medication. When she checks her
blood pressure at home, it is usually normal. The only problem is that
when she is nervous or upset (a frequent problem in elderly people who
live alone), her blood pressure climbs sky high. We found that I could
prescribe enough blood pressure medication to prevent the occasional
blood pressure spikes. But then, when she was not upset, her blood pressure would often be too low, causing her to become dizzy and lighthead-
ed. The solution to this dilemma was to teach Jeannie AH-OM Breath
meditation. Now when her pressure starts to spike, she sits down and
meditates and her blood pressure quickly comes down. Also, now that she
is meditating regularly, she gets upset much less often, which prevents
her blood pressure from spiking in the first place.

Other advice for people with high blood pressure is to avoid excess
salt, caffeine, and over-the-counter decongestant medicines as these all
raise blood pressure. Some people have the so-called white coat syndrome, where their blood pressure shoots up 20 points or more just
from the stress of being in a doctor's office. So, I also advise my hyper-
tensive patients to get a home blood pressure cuff, check their own blood
pressure weekly and bring those readings to their doctor visits. This may
prevent unnecessarily increasing the dose of their blood pressure medication if their readings at home are consistently normal.

TACHYCARDIA AND DYSRHYTHMIA

Tachycardia is the medical name for a resting heartbeat (or pulse) that
is too fast. Dysrhythmia is a medical term that means abnormal or irregular heartbeat. The heartbeat can be slowed down and some forms of
dysrhythmia can be regulated with prescription medications called beta-
blockers. However, this type of treatment might cause the heart to beat
too slowly and cause other side effects such as fatigue, sexual dysfunction, and cold extremities.

Meditation techniques, however, can be effective means for treating some of these heart rhythm problems. In his pioneering studies of the physiologic response to TM, Herbert Benson demonstrated the heartbeat is slowed by an average of three beats per minute during meditation. The observation that meditation is associated with a slowing of the heart rate was also found in the previously cited study done by Vernon Barnes. A randomized clinical trial by Jane Leserman and colleagues (including Herbert Benson) from the Harvard Medical School studied twenty-seven patients undergoing cardiac surgery. The meditation method they used in the study is called the Relaxation Response (see page 47 for instructions). The patients in the group randomized to practice meditation had a statistically significant lower incidence of a tachycardia syndrome called supraventricular tachycardia compared to the control group. Another clinical trial led by Dr. Benson, published in the journal *Lancet,* studied patients with coronary artery disease who practiced the Relaxation Response for twenty minutes twice daily. After four weeks, a reduced frequency of the dysrhythmia called premature ventricular contractions (PVCs) was documented in eight of eleven patients studied.

One of my patients, Jim, is a semi-retired, former police officer. Jim still does consulting work in the field of disaster preparedness. He had recently received offers to consult on a big project in Japan and to teach a series of classes on disaster preparedness at a local university. Jim was obviously proud to still be able to help his community with his professional expertise, but he was worried that taking on these new challenges would be too much for him. Jim has a past history of heart bypass surgery and already was taking a beta-blocker medicine for his blood pressure.

Jim came to see me when he was experiencing a feeling of a faster heartbeat (tachycardia) and a sensation of palpitations associated with an irregular pulse. Jim looked anxious, but his physical exam was fine except for slightly elevated blood pressure. An electrocardiogram (EKG) revealed an occasional PVC, but was otherwise normal. I ordered a screening cardiac stress test, which also turned out to be normal. I then recommended that Jim try meditation to reduce his stress and to see if it would help reduce his blood pressure and palpitations. Jim came to the meditation classes where he learned AH-OM Breath meditation, and he took to meditation like a duck takes to water. His palpitations and PVCs stopped, and his blood pressure returned to normal. Jim went ahead with his new professional projects and remains happy and proud of his consulting and teaching work.

HEART ATTACK

Heart attack, also called myocardial infarction, is one of the most devastating medical problems a person can encounter. It can cause sudden death or render someone a "cardiac cripple" from a serious heart muscle weakness known as cardiomyopathy. Due to cardiomyopathy, a person might experience terrible shortness of breath caused by their lungs filling up with fluid, a condition called congestive heart failure.

In 2007, Ravi Jayadevappa and fellow researchers at the University of Pennsylvania reported a randomized control trial of twenty-three African Americans with congestive heart failure, who were randomized to either a TM or a health education group. This six-month-long study found that TM resulted in improved exercise capacity and feeling of well-being in patients with congestive heart failure. Also, the TM group had fewer hospitalizations during the study period.

An eight-month study of twenty-one patients with coronary artery disease by J.W. Zamarra and associates, published in the *American Journal of Cardiology,* found that patients taught TM had a 14.7 percent improvement in treadmill stress test performance compared to the control group.

My patient Rick is a retired dermatology physician. After retirement, Rick had gotten pleasure from delving into alternative methods of healing, including taking courses in shamanism and herbalism. Rick had a high blood cholesterol level, but he was afraid of possible side effects from the statin drugs that are usually prescribed to treat high cholesterol. He figured that taking herbal supplements would be a better way to lower his high cholesterol level. Unfortunately, the supplements, along with attention to proper diet, made very little difference to Rick's cholesterol level. Rick also had occasional vague feelings of chest discomfort, which we later found out was due to recurrent episodes of angina.

After Rick started coming to meditation class, he began to overcome his fear of taking medication to treat his high cholesterol. He started taking a prescription statin drug, which normalized his cholesterol level without any side effects. About the same time, Rick allowed me to order a cardiac exercise stress test. The results were dangerously abnormal. An angiogram showed that all three of his major coronary arteries were severely narrowed and nearly completely obstructed with cholesterol-containing plaque. Rick eventually underwent a successful triple-vessel heart bypass surgery, and his follow-up cardiac stress tests have all been normal. Rick is still leading a very active and vigorous lifestyle. He often travels the world taking part in alternative healing workshops and teaching some of his own health workshops.

Mack is another of my patients who recently underwent treatment of his angina with coronary angioplasty, a procedure that uses a balloon catheter to open clogged coronary arteries. Afterward, he began feeling depressed, which commonly follows angioplasty or bypass surgery as these patients begin to fear their mortality. Mack took my meditation class and learned AH-OM Breath meditation and about meditating on The Five Remembrances and walking meditation (both described in Chapter 4). He has now come to terms with accepting his mortality, and he is no longer depressed nor constantly fearful he is about to die. More importantly, he is now spending more time enjoying the wonders of life that are still available to him in the present moment, like walking outdoors and being with his wife and grandchildren.

Another effective treatment plan for reversing heart disease for patients like Mack and Rick has been devised by cardiologist Dean Ornish. Dr. Ornish has shown that a lifestyle modification program of regular meditation, vegetarian diet, smoking cessation, and exercise can very successfully stop the buildup of cholesterol and plaque in coronary arteries. Dr. Ornish, in a clinical trial published in 1990 in the journal *Lancet,* has even demonstrated that some of his patients experience a dissolving (regression) of the atherosclerotic plaques that had been obstructing blood flow through their coronary arteries.

Leslie has been my patient for many years. She had shockingly witnessed her husband die within minutes of suddenly collapsing on their living-room floor from a massive heart attack. Leslie, who herself had

had quadruple coronary bypass surgery, was living with the fear that a similar fate could befall her. She is also very overweight, which aggravates her severe reflux esophagitis (heartburn), making assessment of her periodic chest pains tricky. On top of all that stress, Leslie supports her ailing elderly mother, single daughter, and two small grandchildren, all of whom live with her, by continuing to hold down a full-time job at a large retail department store. She often missed work with many office visits to her cardiologist and her gastroenterologist, punctuated by trips to the emergency room to evaluate chest pains.

When she was much younger, Leslie had learned Vipassana Meditation, which uses awareness of breath as the main focus for meditation. After her bypass surgery, Leslie had tried to resume a regular meditation practice to cope with all her stress, anxiety, and depression. But she found it was too difficult to stay concentrated and soon stopped practicing. Then Leslie learned the AH-OM Breath meditation technique, which combines an internally chanted mantra sound with awareness of breath. The addition of the mantra sound to awareness of breath as a focus for her meditation worked much better than just focusing on her breath alone, because it became easier for Leslie to stay concentrated and avoid lapsing into thinking. With regular meditation practice, Leslie was able to transform her fear, anger, and sadness. She was able to stop dwelling in the past or worrying about the future. Instead, she could spend more time feeling peace and happiness in the present moment. Leslie gained insight that her chest pains were usually simple heartburn and not a reason to panic or despair.

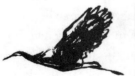

CHRONIC FATIGUE SYNDROME

From time to time, many people experience occasional tiredness or a general lack of energy. Chronic fatigue syndrome is a much more disabling form of persistent and severe tiredness, not associated with any other illness, which lasts uninterrupted for many months or years. It disrupts a person's capacity to work, socialize, or enjoy life. This is a condition of unknown (probably multifactorial) cause. It is possible some cases may be a result of a previous viral infection, like Epstein-Barr virus (the virus that causes mono-nucleosis), or be a manifestation of depression or chronic drug or alcohol abuse. But usually no specific reason can be found for this disabling syndrome.

If a doctor invented a pill that could safely boost a person's energy level, that doctor would surely be an overnight billionaire. But no such safe and effective "energy pill" yet exists. However, the regular practice of meditation is associated with an increase in a person's energy level and in their level of attention and awareness. Meditation is a safe and effective treatment, which I have seen help several patients with chronic fatigue become more energetic, happy, and productive. Movement meditation, such as walking meditation (page 105), the Chinese movement and stretching exercises called t'ai chi, or qi gong, can also very effectively supplement sitting meditation to stimulate improved energy levels, muscular endurance, and cardiovascular fitness.

A randomized controlled trial of chronic fatigue syndrome patients by Suraway and associates found that the meditation techniques of Mindfulness-Based Stress Reduction combined with mindfulness-based cognitive therapy significantly improved levels of fatigue and physical functioning in these people.

Colleen was an energetic, artistic woman with long red hair and deeply green eyes, who owned her own fashion-design company as well as ran a little antique store. At age forty-one, over a period of several weeks, she experienced a severe decline in her energy level that progressed to the point that she could no longer keep up her former energetic pace. She tried to boost her energy by drinking a lot of coffee. But she was still too tired to run a business, and had to give up her design company and sell her antique store.

By the time I saw her, Colleen had sought help from a variety of doctors, naturopaths, and herbalists looking for a "magic" energy-pill cure. She had been tried on antidepressants, antianxiety drugs, Chinese herbs, special diets, and anti-yeast treatments. But none of these treatments made a difference to her chronic fatigue.

A few weeks before her fatigue began, she had had a two-week long flu-like illness. But the blood tests I ordered showed no evidence of an ongoing, active infection (including Epstein-Barr virus), and no organ system dysfunction or other metabolic disturbance such as thyroid disease or hypoglycemia. Colleen did not use alcohol or illegal drugs, nor did she seem clinically depressed (only frustrated with her persistent tiredness), and brain scans and other neurological tests were normal.

Colleen eventually started a daily meditation practice using a combination of both AH-OM Breath meditation and walking meditation, along with doing regular stretching and stationary bicycle exercises, eating a sensible diet, and not drinking so much coffee. Very soon after beginning that program, she stopped worrying about the future and regretting the past. She started to feel less frustrated and more accepting of her life, and she again began to enjoy making new drawings for clothes designs. She slowly also began to recover her energy. Colleen then started an Internet-based antique sales business, which is now quite successful.

GASTROINTESTINAL PROBLEMS

Stomach ulcer and gastritis, heartburn (gastroesophageal reflux disease), irritable bowel syndrome, ulcerative colitis, and Crohn's disease are common gastrointestinal conditions that can be helped by meditation, because they are often caused by or exacerbated by stress and anxiety.

STOMACH ULCER AND GASTRITIS

Brian is a high-powered salesman for a big wholesale company. The pressure to make good on his sales accounts was constantly causing a high output of acid to be produced in his stomach and a frequent painful, burning sensation in his upper abdomen. He had an endoscopy and was found to have a stomach ulcer (an erosion in the lining of his stomach), as well as a diffusely inflamed stomach lining (gastritis). Medication was prescribed to reduce the acid production and help heal the damage. After six weeks of treatment, Brian was taken off the medication and felt well for a while. Then the old pattern of work stress associated with upper abdominal pain recurred. During an office visit, I introduced Brian to the meditation exercise called The Stress Reliever, described in

Chapter 4 (page 148). I also gave him a printed copy of the instructions to take home and practice once or twice a day. Brian soon became better able to handle his stress. He developed a different perspective on his work responsibilities and attendant time pressures. His abdominal pain stopped and he has been able to stay off medication since.

It is also important for people with a history of gastritis or ulcer disease to avoid all over-the-counter anti-inflammatory drugs (like aspirin and ibuprofen), minimize intake of alcohol and caffeine, and cease any cigarette smoking.

HEARTBURN

Heartburn (also called gastroesophageal reflux disease or GERD) is an irritation of the esophagus that is made worse by stress-induced overproduction of stomach acid. In the journal *Gastroenterology,* J. McDonald-Haile and associates reported a controlled study of twenty subjects who had esophageal reflux disease, which found that relaxation training resulted in significantly fewer reflux symptoms. In the study, all patients had symptoms and acid levels checked before and after a stressful task such as solving math problems. Half of the study group was instructed in a progressive muscular relaxation exercise to try to relax each muscle group in sequence, while repeating the word "relax" with their out-breath. The control group attended a health education class on causes and treatments for GERD. Compared to the control group, the muscle relaxation group had two-thirds less acid formation, and greater than a 50 percent reduction in symptoms of acid reflux.

The progressive muscular relaxation intervention in the study above is very similar to the "body scan" portion of two of the meditation exercises described in Chapter 4, Buddha's Breathing Exercises and Meditation on the Whole Person. Doing these types of meditation exercises would, therefore, also be expected to reduce the severity of heartburn symptoms in many people with GERD.

Certain foods also make heartburn worse. It helps to minimize intake of chocolate, fatty and fried foods, citrus juices and carbonated beverages, and any foods that are found to aggravate the symptoms, and avoid excess weight gain or laying flat right after a meal.

IRRITABLE BOWEL SYNDROME

Irritable bowel syndrome (IBS) is another condition that is very stress sensitive. Teresa is a twenty-nine-year-old sales executive who has the responsibility and stress of managing the work of a lot of employees. She came to me with a history of having frequent symptoms of alternating constipation and diarrhea and an uncomfortable bloating pain in her belly off and on for years. She would miss days at work due to these symptoms of IBS.

Teresa was prescribed a combination of a high-fiber diet, regular exercise, and meditation. I taught her the AH-OM Breath meditation to calm her mind and the pain-reducing meditation techniques described in the Chapter 4 section "Meditations for Transforming Pain." When her belly hurt, Teresa would imagine she was breathing in and out through a hole in her belly button, and she would also imagine that the pain was easing more with each out-breath. The meditation practice called Mindfulness of Eating, described in Chapter 4 on page 140, can also help digestion and reduce the pain and bloating of IBS. After she learned these meditation and dietary practices, Teresa's IBS symptoms calmed down to a rare, minor inconvenience.

A clinical trial conducted by Laurie Keefer and fellow researchers, published in *Behaviour Research and Therapy*, followed ten patients with IBS for one year. The participants were taught to do Relaxation Response meditation. The study found that, after three months, these patients had significant improvements in flatulence, belching, bloating, and diarrhea. And these improvements lasted for more than a year after the meditation training.

ULCERATIVE COLITIS AND CROHN'S DISEASE

Ulcerative colitis and Crohn's disease are two forms of severe inflammation of the intestinal tract, producing abdominal pain, bloody diarrhea, and mucus in the stools. The cause of these two chronic diseases is unknown. But it is known that stress in these patients may precipitate an acute flare-up of inflammatory colitis.

In a randomized clinical trial published in *Pain*, L. Shaw and A. Ehrlich

Toyko Ghoul

Ring

Wish

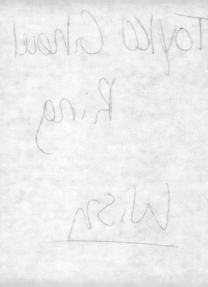

studied twenty people with ulcerative colitis. Half the study patients were randomized to a progressive muscle relaxation intervention; along with a control group, they were followed for six weeks. The relaxation group with ulcerative colitis had significantly fewer pain episodes and less pain intensity, and they used less of the anti-inflammatory pain medications than the control group. Hence, it would be reasonable for people with colitis to try practicing meditation to reduce pain severity and frequency.

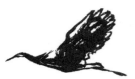 ## INFECTIOUS DISEASES

We all possess the innate ability to help protect ourselves from infectious disease. This wondrous infectious disease prevention system is called the immune system. There is now scientific evidence that the regular practice of meditation can boost immune system function.

In a randomized clinical trial of forty-one participants published in *Psychosomatic Medicine* (2003), Drs. Richard Davidson and Jon Kabat-Zinn and associates studied antibody levels in meditators and non-meditators after receiving a flu shot. The meditation group participants were taught Mindfulness-Based Stress Reduction by Dr. Kabat-Zinn, which took place weekly, for two and a half to three hours, over a six-week period. All study participants were then vaccinated with the influenza vaccine (flu shot). The study measured anti-influenza antibodies at four and eight weeks after vaccination. They found that the meditators displayed a significantly greater (two times greater) rise in their levels of anti-influenza antibodies.

Other research studies have demonstrated that meditation is associated with positive effects on the immune system. The Bakke study, previously cited, demonstrated that a type of guided meditation was associated with increases in blood levels of natural killer white blood cells that are known to be important in fighting viral infections as well as cancer. The other previously cited study (in cancer patients) by Dr. Lengacher's group found that the natural killer white blood cells of patients who practiced guided meditation were found to have an enhanced capacity for cytotoxicity (virus- and cancer-cell-killing ability).

Taken together, these three research studies are evidence that meditation practice can result in a more vigorous immune system. Importantly, stress has been shown to decrease immune system function. Since meditation reduces stress, this is yet another mechanism by which meditation can help to prevent infection or speed recovery from infection.

There are probably multiple pathways whereby meditation, by causing changes in brain activity, could potentially influence the performance of the immune system. The brain connects to the endocrine system by way of the hypothalamus and pituitary gland located deep in the base of the brain, and through the autonomic (sympathetic/parasympathetic) nervous system connecting directly to the adrenal glands and pancreas. Altogether, this is called the neuroendocrine system. A medical review article in *Cellular Immunology* (2008) entitled "Neuroendocrine Factors Alter Host Defense by Modulating Immune Function" discusses the effects of this interaction. It states, "Crosstalk between the neuroendocrine and immune systems can also result in production of factors by the nervous and endocrine systems that alter immune cell function and subsequent modulation of immune responses against infectious agents and other pathogens."

COMMON COMMUNITY-ACQUIRED INFECTIONS

The most common types of infections seen in my medical practice are upper respiratory infections and viral intestinal infections. A person with an upper respiratory infection may have a fever, bad sore throat, nasal congestion, and heavy cough. A viral intestinal infection might cause nausea, vomiting, diarrhea, and abdominal pain.

When this happens to someone, there is often a psychological feeling of despair that sets in. How often have you heard someone with a bad case of the flu say something like "Woe is me. I feel like I'm gonna die"? While meditation doesn't replace the need for antibiotics to treat bacterial infections, meditation can reverse the feeling of despair and replace it with a calm sense of confidence in eventual recovery. In these circumstances, I recommend practicing the exercise called Meditation on the Whole Person (page 119). In addition to probably enhancing the immune system, this meditation exercise can also remind an ailing patient that there is so much more to their whole person than the infection they are fighting. This can restore a feeling of well-being and optimism about their eventual recovery.

HIV/AIDS

Infection with the human immunodeficiency virus (HIV) can lead to acquired immunodeficiency syndrome (AIDS), a condition in which the immune system begins to weaken, leading to life-threatening opportunistic infections. People living with HIV/AIDS infection often have difficulty with quality-of-life issues. A randomized, controlled trial conducted by researchers at Yale University School of Medicine looked at meditation and massage used in the treatment of advanced HIV/AIDS patients. They studied fifty-eight people with late-stage AIDS who listened to a Metta meditation audiocassette and got a daily massage for one month. (In Metta meditation, also called Loving-Kindness meditation, one focuses awareness on repeating a positive healing sentiment such as "May I be safe, know peace, and be healthy and happy.") This clinical study by Anna-Leila Williams and colleagues concluded, "The combination of meditation and massage has a significantly favorable influence on overall and spiritual quality of life in late-stage disease relative to standard care."

Jill Bormann and associates at the Veteran's Administration in San Diego conducted a randomized, controlled trial of ninety-three patients to assess the effects of a stress-management strategy using a mantra on HIV outcomes. This clinical study used a mantra-type meditation technique that consisted of patients silently repeating a phrase of their own choosing that had spiritual connotations. And they went to group meetings that taught things such as practicing one-pointed attention by repeating a mantra, or intentionally slowing down and mindfully engaging in one task at a time. The control group also went to educational group classes and viewed home videotapes of material related to treatments for HIV. Over the ten-week study period, the mantra group improved significantly more than the control group at reducing anger and increasing spiritual connectedness, as measured by standard psychological tests. The investigators concluded this type of mantra-based meditation can help in managing psychological distress and enhancing existential spiritual well-being in adults living with HIV/AIDS.

A case in point is my patient Diane. Diane is a thirty-nine-year-old real estate agent. She came to see me when other doctors were unable to diagnose the cause of a chronic cough. My physical exam revealed enlarged liver, spleen, and lymph nodes. A high-resolution computerized axial tomography (CAT or CT) scan of her lungs also showed enlarged lymph nodes inside her chest. Further evaluation demonstrated she had a rare lung infection with *Mycobacterium avium,* an organism that usually does not cause human infection. This led to a positive antibody test for the HIV virus, which causes AIDS.

Diane was, of course, psychologically devastated. When we discussed how she might have gotten the HIV virus, she recalled that five years earlier she had gotten a divorce after she had found out that her husband was having a homosexual relationship with his former roommate who, it turns out, had AIDS. Diane was referred for treatment to the nearby university AIDS clinic that started her on an AIDS treatment "cocktail" of several drugs. With treatment she began to recover, and the numbers of her T cells, white blood cells crucial for preventing infection, rose. But it was meditation and participation in group therapy that restored her psychological and emotional balance. She was then able to accept the diagnosis of AIDS in a way that allowed her to go on with her job at the real estate office and be able to smile.

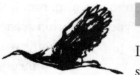

INSOMNIA

Insomnia is a very common complaint in patients seeking help from their family doctor. It is impossible to feel fresh in the morning without adequate sleep. Despite the fact that we do have medications that can induce sleep, chronic insomnia remains a vexing disorder to treat. This is because sleep medications can cause unpleasant side effects; they are habit forming; and their use does not produce a normal type of sleep. I have found music therapy CDs can help some patients to fall back asleep naturally. Unfortunately, however, this doesn't work for most patients. On the other hand, a calming meditation like AH-OM Breath, practiced while lying in bed, usually does help most people fall back into a natural, restful sleep.

The randomized controlled trial conducted by Linda Carlson and associates with breast and prostate cancer patients, mentioned earlier, found a significant improvement in the quality of sleep in the group of cancer patients who were trained in Mindfulness-Based Stress Reduction meditation.

A controlled clinical trial of twenty people with sleep-onset insomnia was done at Harvard Medical School by G. D. Jacobs and six coinvestigators, including Herbert Benson. They found that adding training in Relaxation Response meditation, as part of a behavior modification treatment for insomniacs, resulted in a 77 percent improvement in the time to sleep onset compared to the control group.

Steve, a twenty-five-year-old U.S. Navy Corpsman, recently came to my meditation class because he couldn't stay asleep at night. He often would wake in the middle of the night and start thinking about his stressful day at work. After taking the first meditation class and learning about AH-OM Breath meditation, Steve returned the next week and declared to the class that the technique "was awesome." It helped him return to sleep faster and stay asleep longer.

To learn how you can use this and other specific meditation techniques to treat insomnia, see the section in Chapter 4 entitled "Meditations for a Good Night's Sleep."

LUNG AND RESPIRATORY DISORDERS

Included here are the problems of asthma, chronic obstructive pulmonary disease, and hyperventilation syndrome.

ASTHMA

Asthma causes obstruction of airflow in the lungs due to both constriction of the bronchial tubes and thick mucus plugs within the bronchial tubes. A severe asthma attack is one of the scariest feelings there is, because the victim's wind is suddenly cut off and they may feel as if they are about to die. This horrible feeling of suffocation was what Brandon experienced almost every time his asthma was triggered. One of the commonest triggers of his asthma was anxiety and stress. After Brandon started practicing AH-OM Breath meditation, the frequency of his asthma attacks dramatically decreased. We also discussed avoiding environmental triggers (listed below). While Brandon still has an occasional asthma attack, they are now much less severe and less scary for him.

In order to investigate the effect of one type of meditation on patients with moderate to severe asthma, a double-blind, randomized controlled trial of fifty-nine people with asthma was published in *Thorax* by Ramesh Manocha and associates at the Royal Hospital for Women in Sydney, Australia. The intervention of Sahaja Yoga meditation demonstrated short-term improvement in lung function in patients with poorly controlled asthma. Sahaja Yoga is a system of meditation based on yoga principles, which aims at helping a person learn to maintain a period of "thoughtless awareness" or "mental silence" in which the meditator is fully alert and aware. The meditators were asked to practice for ten to twenty minutes twice daily, and repeat measurements were taken after four months and again after six months. The control group practiced more general relaxation exercises for the same periods of time.

The investigators in this study employed a standard experimental method to study asthma patients in which a drug called methacholine is used to induce increased resistance to airflow in the lungs of the test subjects. The results of this study found that at four months the asthma patients in the meditation group had far less airway resistance when given methacholine than the control group. Unfortunately, however, when retested two months later, the decreased airway hyperresponsiveness of the meditation group to methacholine did not persist. (It should, however, be pointed out that the control group was using relaxation exercises, which could also have had a meditation-like effect.)

Avoiding environmental triggers like smoke, dust, and (for some people) pollens and pet dander are other important non-medication ways to reduce asthma. For people who have exercise-induced asthma, staying well hydrated and avoiding heavy exercise on very dry or dusty days can help prevent asthma attacks. Also, during cold and flu season, asthmatics should try to avoid getting respiratory infections, which can trigger asthma, by avoiding doing things like shaking hands with people who are ill, or sitting next to someone with an obvious cold in a crowded airplane or bus. As mentioned earlier in the section on infectious disease, the Davidson–Kabat-Zinn study showed that meditation can boost the immune response to a flu shot. So, it may be that meditation can lower the risk of influenza-induced asthma in people who have received the flu vaccine.

CHRONIC OBSTRUCTIVE PULMONARY DISEASE

Chronic obstructive pulmonary disease (COPD), also called emphysema and chronic bronchitis is usually a disease of cigarette smokers. This devastating and insidious illness slowly takes your breath away and eventually renders its victims permanently tied to an oxygen tank and feeling terrible. So, if you smoke, try to quit at all costs, as the lung damage is ongoing. Unfortunately, after a person quits, the damage that was done never totally heals. AH-OM Breath meditation can help someone cope with the anxiety and depression that frequently accompanies this illness. (See also the section "Mood and Affective Disorders.")

For this chronic respiratory disease, as well as for people with recurrent asthma, I recommend being mindful of your lungs and calming yourself by practicing Buddha's Breathing Exercises on page 114. Also described in that Chapter 4 is the diaphragmatic breathing technique called the Yoga Complete Breath (page 116). Practicing this breathing technique along with purse-lipped exhalation can improve respiratory capacity in people with COPD. One of my COPD patients said the meditation breathing exercises helped her regain some sense of control over her breath, and walking meditation helped her improve her exercise capacity.

HYPERVENTILATION SYNDROME

Hyperventilation syndrome is a situation where a person uncontrollably breathes too rapidly. This is often triggered by a psychological panic attack. Natasha suffered from hyperventilation attacks that left her feeling dizzy, with lips and fingers tingling, chest hurting, and a panicky feeling that her throat was closing off and she was about to pass out. These upsetting symptoms frequently compelled Natasha to go to the hospital emergency room for evaluation. Learning to meditate using Buddha's Breathing Exercises has allowed Natasha to minimize her panic attacks and hyperventilation and avoid visits to the local ER.

MENOPAUSAL SYMPTOMS AND PREMENSTRUAL SYNDROME

J. H. Irvin, from Harvard Medical School, and associates published a randomized controlled trial of 103 postmenopausal women in the *Journal of Psychosomatic Obstetrics and Gynecology.* They studied the use of the meditation technique known as the Relaxation Response to treat women with menopausal symptoms who were not on hormone replacement therapy. The study included a control group of women who were told to read leisure material for twenty minutes daily. The meditation group of women were given instructions on how to elicit the relaxation response (see Dr. Benson's instructions for this technique on the following page) and given a twenty-minute tape for home use to practice daily for seven weeks. The investigators found the Relaxation Response group had statistically significant reductions in intensity of hot flashes, anxiety, and depression; there were no changes in the control group.

This information about treating menopausal symptoms with meditation seems much more important now than at the time it was published in 1996. This is because, since that study was published, medical research has proven that what used to be the mainstay of treatment for this disorder—hormone replacement therapy—has now been proven to increase a woman's risk of heart attack, stroke, and breast cancer.

Six years earlier at Harvard Medical School, Herbert Benson and colleagues Goodale and Domar supervised a randomized controlled trial of the effect of Relaxation Response training for women experiencing symptoms of premenstrual syndrome (PMS). This study involved forty-six women assigned randomly to one of three groups. One control group just charted their symptoms. Another group was told to sit quietly and read leisure material of their own choice for fifteen to twenty minutes twice a day. The third group was told to practice the Relaxation Response for fifteen to twenty minutes twice daily.

The test subjects rated themselves for specific physical symptoms like cramps, general physical discomfort, water retention, and fatigue, as well as for emotional symptoms like lability of mood, anger, anxiety, and social withdrawal. The results of this three-month trial, published in the *Journal of Obstetrics and Gynecology*, found a highly statistically significant reduction in both physical and emotional PMS symptoms in the group randomized to practice the Relaxation Response. And the women with the most severe PMS symptoms responded with the most improvement.

RELAXATION RESPONSE MEDITATION

This simple mantra-based meditative technique was pioneered in the United States by Harvard cardiologist Herbert Benson more than thirty years ago. The technique, used by Dr. Benson in many of his groundbreaking studies and introduced to the general public in his 1975 best seller *The Relaxation Response,* is easy to describe and do:

1. Sit quietly in a comfortable position with your eyes closed.

2. Deeply relax all your muscles, beginning with your face and progressing down to your feet.

3. Breathe through your nose, becoming aware of your breath. As you breathe out, say the word "one" silently to yourself.

4. Do not worry whether you are successful at achieving a deep level of relaxation. Maintain a passive attitude and permit relaxation to occur at its own pace. When a distracting thought comes to mind, simply say to yourself, "Oh well," and go back to the word "one." Try this for ten to twenty minutes a day.

MOOD AND AFFECTIVE DISORDERS

This next category of conditions includes anxiety, depression, and other mood disorders such as loneliness, despair, intermittent sadness, stress-related nervousness, and panic attacks. Meditation can be helpful in the prevention and treatment of these forms of emotional suffering. If these mood disorders persist over a long time, they can have a direct adverse impact on a person's physical health.

HEALTH EFFECTS OF NEGATIVE AND POSITIVE EMOTIONS

Medical studies have consistently found that people who suffer from the negative emotion of prolonged depression are more likely to have ill health and a shorter life span. In 1999 B. W. Penninx and colleagues published a study in the *Archives of General Psychiatry* that followed a group of 3,056 men and women for four years. After adjusting for socio-demographics, health status, and health behaviors, depression was associated with a 1.83 greater risk of dying. A clinical study published by M. Ganguli and associates in *Archives of General Psychiatry* in 2002 also found depression to be a predictor of increased mortality rates. A 1995 study by neuroscientist G. M. Gilad at the Technion-Israel Institute of Technology, published in *Mechanisms of Ageing and Development,* investigated the negative consequences of chronic stress in rats. This study found that the life span of rodents is inversely related to the intensity of their behavioral and neuroendocrine responses to stressful stimuli.

In a 2003 study by John F. Todaro and colleagues, published in the *American Journal of Cardiology,* participants with the highest levels of negative emotions experienced the greatest incidence of coronary heart disease. H. D. Sesso and coinvestigators published a study in the *American Journal of Cardiology* of 1,305 men and found that, over the seven-year study, men with depression were approximately 50 to 75 percent more likely to develop coronary heart disease. A 2006 study from the Harvard School of Public Health published in the *Annals of Behavioral*

Medicine found anxiety also increased the risk of developing coronary heart disease.

From the studies cited above, it is clear that negative emotional states like depression, anxiety, and chronic stress have a negative impact on physical health. The medical literature also contains research studies investigating the health benefits of positive emotions. There have been several large studies published in the medical literature investigating the health consequences of being a happy person with an optimistic outlook on life.

A Yale University research survey conducted by B. R. Levy and fellow researchers followed 660 people aged fifty or more over a twenty-three-year period. That study found that people with a positive self-perception of aging lived an average of seven and a half years longer than those with a less positive self-perception of aging.

A study by E. J. Gilray and associates, published in the *Archives of General Psychiatry* (2004), followed ninety-four elderly people aged sixty-five to eighty-five over a nine-year period. This study adjusted for age, sex, chronic disease, education, smoking, alcohol consumption, history of cardiovascular disease or hypertension, body mass index, and total cholesterol level. After adjusting for all these risk factors, the researchers found that, compared to subjects with a high level of pessimism, those reporting a high level of optimism had a 45 percent lower death rate from all causes and a 77 percent lower death rate from cardiovascular disease.

Other recent comparable clinical studies that focused on whether happiness and optimism affected death risk came to similar conclusions. Data from the famous six-decade-long Nun Study, reported by Deborah Danner and investigators in the *Journal of Personality and Social Psychology* (2001), found that the happiest quartile of nuns in early adulthood lived an average of 6.9 years longer than the unhappiest quartile of nuns. A study of 839 people reported in the *Mayo Clinic Proceedings* in 2000 also found a pessimistic style, as measured by the Optimism-Pessimism Scale of the Minnesota Multiphasic Personality Inventory, was significantly associated with increased mortality rate. H. Iwasa and associates published in *Nippon Ronen Igakkai Zasshi (Japanese Journal of Geriatrics)* a seven-year study of 2,447 men and women aged fifty-two to seventy-seven years. They found that there was a "significant and independent association between a low level of subjective well-being and the risk for all-cause mortality in both genders." They concluded, "Satisfaction with life is an important factor affecting longevity among middle-aged and elderly people."

In addition to the risk of death, another subject of investigation is the association between nonfatal medical illness and optimism versus pessimism. A study published in the *Journal of Personality and Social Psychology* in 1988 by C. Peterson and colleagues followed ninety-four Harvard graduates, aged thirty to sixty years, over a thirty-five-year study period. They found that, even when physical and mental health at age twenty-five was controlled for, pessimism in early adulthood was an independent risk factor for poor health in middle and late adulthood. A study by M. F. Scheier and associates, reported in a 1999 *Archives of Internal Medicine,* looked at 3,019 patients undergoing coronary artery bypass graft surgery. They found that compared to pessimistic people, optimistic people were about twice as likely to have a good surgical outcome and avoid complications like heart attack, wound infection, or the need to be rehospitalized for repeat bypass surgery of coronary angioplasty. The study authors concluded, "Fostering positive expectations may promote better recovery."

From the above-referenced medical studies, it is quite clear that being basically a happy person has a positive impact on a person's susceptibility to illness and chances for living a long (and happy) life.

MINOR DEPRESSION

Pete is a retired electronics engineer in his eighties. Pete is partially balding, a little pudgy, likes to wear baggy clothes, and grins a lot. In fact, he looks a little like a jovial Captain Kangaroo. He and I share a common interest in brain science. Usually when I see Pete we have an animated discussion about the latest book by Antonio Damassio or Vilayanur Ramachandran, or one of the other bright lights in the field of neuroscience. Pete is also very kind and compassionate toward his five-year-old grandson, Joey, who loves to hug people, but who is also blind and has Down's syndrome. Pete often takes Joey to the park, or just plays with his "special little guy" on the floor.

At one point, when Joey had lost most of his sight and his future seemed bleak, Pete became depressed and lost his appetite for food and life. He began having frequent stomachaches, insomnia, tiredness, and felt sad most of the time, but at no time did he contemplate suicide. I persuaded Pete to come to a meditation class. He thought he knew what meditation was all about—he thought it was a form of deep thinking. What he found, to his surprise, was that meditation occurred during an absence of thinking. This was a fascinating revelation to him and he began practicing AH-OM Breath meditation and walking meditation on a regular basis.

Meditation enabled Pete to better appreciate what he still had in the present, including his wondrous little grandson. Pete stopped worrying so much about what might happen in the future to little Joey, and soon Pete started having fun with his grandson again. His depression lifted, his abdominal pain stopped, and his appetite and sleep pattern improved. Pete is now his old ebullient self again, and is still getting joy out of exploring the frontiers of neuroscience at age eighty-two.

MAJOR DEPRESSION

Many people with serious depression completely lose the ability to concentrate. This makes meditation impossible for them. For any severely depressed person with a major clinical depression or bipolar manic-depressive illness, the most important intervention is prescription anti-depressant medication. This can restore the normal brain levels of certain neurotransmitters that are necessary to ward off depression. Later, when the person with depression has improved, and he or she can concentrate again, meditation may play a useful role in an integrative approach to the treatment and prevention of depression.

Take Harry for example. Harry is a sixty-three-year-old who retired early from his plumbing business due to being disabled from a back injury and depression. He had attempted suicide at age fifty-one, but years later he was feeling much better and stopped taking his antidepressant medication. As a younger man he had learned a Tibetan meditation technique, but stopped his meditation practice in his early forties when his plumbing business had become very busy.

When Harry came to see me as a patient a couple of years ago, he had been seriously depressed for several months. He constantly felt sad and blue. He woke up most nights at 3:00 A.M. and couldn't get back to sleep. He dreaded getting out of bed in the morning, and after he finally dragged himself out of bed he had no energy to do anything. He also had no appetite for food and had lost twenty pounds. Harry lost all desire for sex or intimacy with his wife. He didn't want to call or visit with friends or other family members, so he just moped around the house all day long. His memory was slipping because he couldn't concentrate on what other people told him, so he worried he might be getting Alzheimer's disease. Harry felt hopeless and helpless and wasn't sure if life was worth living anymore. He had started thinking suicidal thoughts, but he had no specific plan for how he might attempt suicide.

After deeply and sympathetically listening to his story, the next thing I tried to do to help Harry was to prescribe a starting dose of an antidepressant medication, and at the same time referred him to an excellent psychiatrist. The psychiatrist later increased the dose of the medication and eventually added a second medication. After a few weeks, Harry started to get his appetite and energy back, and began to feel that life was worth living again. He also recovered his ability to concentrate, so I then suggested he try resuming his Tibetan meditation practice. This practice further restored Harry's self-confidence, as well as his ability to enjoy spending time with his friends and family and his capacity to express his love for his wife.

This clinical case points out how valuable it can be to integrate traditional medication therapy with complementary methods like meditation in healing the mind, body, and spirit. I think it would have been dangerous to try to treat Harry with meditation alone, as that likely would not have worked and would have exposed him to a serious risk of suicide. To avoid that grave outcome, a person with a major depression must be evaluated by a qualified physician as part of a comprehensive plan for management and follow-up.

SADNESS

A number of recent studies in the medical literature have found that clinical depression is often overdiagnosed in the United States. This leads to the overprescribing of antidepressant medications that alter brain chemistry. Often what is thought to be clinical depression is actually a natural reaction to experiencing the death of a family member, being laid off from a job, or another signal event that produces sadness and grief as a totally appropriate psychological reaction. Deeply listening in an unhurried, nonjudgmental, and supportive way to someone as they tell you their sad story is an important means of helping them heal their grief. These types of sadness, loneliness, or "the blues" are also well treated with meditation techniques, which produce insight and help facilitate a healthy mental healing process.

Sometimes a series of life's little disappointments add up to produce in us a feeling of sadness, frustration, and bitter disappointment. Perhaps you might feel like your friends or family just don't care or understand you; or maybe your car just broke down; or the water pipe on your washing machine busted and flooded your kitchen; or a project at work didn't succeed or seems to be going nowhere; or the electricity went out in your house and you stubbed your toe in the dark trying to find a flashlight. These types of disappointing things occur from time to time in everyone's life. At times, everybody's got "the blues."

In these moments, don't despair or think to yourself, "Why does everything bad happen to me?" Don't look outside yourself for the answer. Instead, look inside yourself, and take refuge in the island of calm and peace within yourself. Just sit down, close your eyes, and calmly pay attention to your in-breath and out-breath. You can use AH-OM Breath meditation, or you might try one of the other meditation techniques described in Chapter 4, such as Meditation on the Whole Person or Buddha's Breathing Exercises. These meditation techniques ease the body, calm painful sensations, and heal negative emotions.

That island of calm and peace is always there inside you. Consider arranging your life in such a way that you can stop your constant "doing," and make time often to go back to that island of peace by practicing meditation. When adversity strikes, even just taking three mindful breaths can do a lot to calm your body and center your mind. This allows you to accept life's inevitable disappointments and restores your feeling of peace, equanimity, and ability to smile again.

ANXIETY

The negative emotion of anxiety can be successfully reduced by the practice of meditation. Jon Kabat-Zinn and researchers working at the University of Massachusetts Stress Reduction Clinic published a 1992 study in the *American Journal of Psychiatry* that showed benefit in using mindfulness meditation to reduce anxiety, panic, and depression. In this study, twenty-two people, who met standard criteria for having generalized anxiety or panic disorder, were taught a type of mindfulness meditation and were studied for three months. Twenty of these subjects experienced significant reductions in anxiety and depression scores. The number of these people who experienced symptoms of panic was also substantially reduced. Some of the mindfulness meditation techniques taught as the Mindfulness-Based Stress Reduction program at the clinic are described in detail in Jon Kabat-Zinn's *Full Catastrophe Living* (Dell Publishing, 1990).

Since the 1992 study noted above, several later studies have been published that show meditation is beneficial in the treatment of anxiety, stress, and some forms of depression and panic attacks. One such randomized controlled trial was published in 2007 in the *Annals of Behavioral Medicine* by Shamini Jain and associates at the University of California Clinical Psychology Program. They compared stress levels in three groups of patients: a control group, another group that received training in mindfulness meditation, and a third group trained in standard relaxation exercises. Both the meditation group and the relaxation group appeared to benefit from the intervention. But the authors also concluded, "Mindfulness meditation may be more specific in its ability to reduce distractive and ruminating thoughts and behaviors."

James Lane and colleagues from the Department of Psychiatry at Duke University Medical Center in Durham, North Carolina, published a study in 2007, in which 133 healthy adults were taught to practice a simple mantra-based meditation technique. They were then assessed to see whether this practice made any difference in their level of stress, anxiety, and negative mood. The test subjects were taught the meditation method in four one-hour classes over a two-week period.

The participants selected for themselves a sound, word, or brief phrase to repeat silently as a mantra for fifteen to twenty minutes twice a day. Their mood was assessed by four different standardized mood scales (Profile of Mood States, Perceived Stress Scale, State-Trait Anxiety Inventory, and Brief Symptom Inventory). The participants' mood was assessed at baseline and at monthly intervals for three months. There was no control group in the study. The results of the study found that compared to baseline, very significant 20 to 40 percent reductions in perceived stress and negative mood were seen at one month, which persisted at the three-month follow-up assessment. Also, frequency of meditation practice made a difference. People who meditated at least once a day scored better than those who meditated less than once a day. The study concluded that "even brief instruction in a simple meditation technique can improve negative mood and perceived stress in healthy adults, which could yield long-term health benefits." This same trend has been reported in many studies (see the bibliography) that look at the beneficial effect of meditation as treatment for mood and affective disorders and stress reduction.

Alessandra is a sixty-eight-year-old woman who grew up in Italy and had been living in California with her Italian-born husband for many years. Alessandra's husband was constantly domineering and verbally abusive to his wife. Alessandra always complained of feeling nervous and anxious, and having other stress-related symptoms like insomnia and tiredness. She knew continuing to live with her husband, who berated her daily for a myriad of minor things, was unhealthy. But she was too afraid to live on her own.

After Alessandra began practicing sitting and walking meditation she was able to see more clearly how toxic her home situation had become. She eventually found the inner strength to make a break with the past and get her own apartment. She started practicing qi gong. She got a dog for companionship, started taking painting classes, and began traveling to visit friends and family back in Italy. She regained her joy of living and felt a liberating sense of freedom. Later, she was even able to forgive her husband for his faults, and be kind and compassionate to him in their new relationship.

STRESS

Almost any illness or symptom of ill health can be associated with stress and fear. The practice of meditation diminishes stress and fear. Therefore, meditation can be a salutary practice for coping with the whole spectrum of human disease and disability.

Stress is an occupational hazard for schoolteachers. A randomized controlled clinical trial investigating the effect of meditation on stress levels in twenty-one secondary-school teachers was published in the journal *Stress Medicine* (1999). In this study by Andrew Winzelberg and Frederic Luskin of the Stanford University Department of Psychiatry and Behavioral Sciences, stress levels were measured with a standard test called the Teacher Stress Inventory at the beginning of the study and again at five weeks and thirteen weeks. In four weekly classes, the meditation group was taught to repeat a mantra, slow down, and practice focusing attention on one thing at a time. These meditation classes were based on the practices taught by Eknath Easwaren in *Meditation: A Simple Eight-Point Program for Translating Spiritual Ideas into Daily Life* (Nilgiri Press, 1978). Winzelberg and Luskin's study found that one week after the end of the four meditation classes the meditation group subjects had been able to significantly reduce their stress levels compared to a control group that had received no classes. However, this difference in stress levels between the two study groups didn't last at an eight-week follow-up assessment.

In the previously mentioned 2007 clinical study by James Lane and associates at Duke University Medical Center, a mantra-based meditation was found to improve negative mood and stress in healthy adults as measured by standardized stress and mood-scoring tests.

One of the meditation exercises used to reduce stress at the University of Massachusetts Stress Reduction Clinic is the body scan. This method is described in detail in *Full Catastrophe Living* by author and clinic director Jon Kabat-Zinn. In short, while lying down, one progressively and consciously relaxes each muscle group in the body. This technique is similar to a meditation exercise practiced at Deer Park and Plum Village Zen monasteries called Total Relaxation. (Plum Village Monastery, home to Thich Nhat Hanh in France, is located fifty-three miles east of Bordeaux.)

One difference is that with Total Relaxation you not only attempt to relax all the muscles of the body, but you also try to visualize and send love and concern to the internal organs such as heart, lungs, liver, intestines, and kidneys.

Dr. Kabat-Zinn has developed a whole series of meditation exercises and stress-reduction classes called Mindfulness-Based Stress Reduction (MBSR). The MBSR classes incorporate many principles of Buddhist philosophy. Dr. Kabat-Zinn has trained quite a few physicians, psychologists, and other people from around the country to teach this method. It is usually taught in a program of eight weekly two-and-a-half to three-hour classes and a full-day retreat. Referring to the University of Massachusetts Stress Reduction Clinic and the program of MBSR in *Full Catastrophe Living,* Dr. Kabat-Zinn writes, "Cultivating mindfulness plays a central role in the changes that the people who come to the stress clinic experience. One way to think of this process of transformation is to think of mindfulness as a lens, taking the scattered and reactive energies of your mind and focusing them into a coherent source of energy for living, for problem solving, and for healing."

Sally, a patient in her forties, is an office manager for a busy ophthalmology practice. She has a teenage son from a previous marriage who is a constant source of stress, and she has a rocky relationship with her boyfriend with whom she lives. Sally came to see me for frequent medical office visits, usually wearing a worried frown on her face. At times she would rush to the hospital emergency room with symptoms of chest pain, palpitations, headaches, and abdominal pains. All the medical evaluations that were done failed to turn up any serious medical illness, and her symptoms appeared to be a manifestation of stress and anxiety.

At a medical office visit, Sally was persuaded to give meditation a try. She started learning to meditate at home by trying the meditation breathing exercise I call The Stress Reliever, described in Chapter 4. The next month she started taking a couple of formal meditation classes and learning to practice mindfulness. Soon Sally was able to relax more at work, deal more effectively with her problems at home, and not to worry so much about what every little symptom meant. She no longer is absent from work due to trips to the ER, and she now comes for follow-up visits with a relaxed smile on her face.

Ben is another example of a patient who received significant stress-reducing benefits from meditation. Ben works as a truck driver and is also a union leader at the company where he works. He suffered tremendous stress from working full-time during the day, and then going to union meetings at night to deal with gut-wrenching union-management disputes. His symptoms were nervousness, fatigue, headaches, and intermittent high blood pressure.

Ben was taught the practice of AH-OM Breath meditation and methods of being mindful during daily activities. He became better able to handle his job stress, and all of his previous stress symptoms quickly resolved. Ben told me mindfulness was, for him, like driving a truck and shifting into a high gear. He said, "You are still traveling along, but you aren't working as hard to get there."

Job stress brought about by conflicts with difficult people at the workplace, and other types of similar conflicts, may produce a lot of anger. Skillfully managing the anger is important to help diminish the harmful effects of this type of stress. See the section entitled "Meditations for Transforming Anger" (page 124) to learn about techniques to help you manage your anger and protect yourself from the adverse effects of this stress.

OBSESSIVE COMPULSIVE DISORDER (OCD)

This is a very distressing psychological disorder that is often difficult to treat. OCD is characterized by intrusive distressing thoughts and repetitive rituals aimed at dislodging those thoughts. Cognitive-behavioral therapy, which aims to modify behavior by helping people change the way they emotionally react to their thoughts, has been used with mixed results showing mild improvement in some OCD patients. In his book *The Mind and the Brain: Neuroplasticity and the Power of Mental Force* (HarperCollins, 2002), psychiatrist Jeffrey M. Schwartz describes using mindfulness techniques to treat patients with OCD. Without using any medication, Dr. Schwartz's treatment technique involves asking his OCD patients to pay attention to their thoughts in a mindful way. Then the OCD patients are asked to substitute a positive thought or behavior for the maladaptive compulsive thought or behavior. In uncontrolled, non-randomized studies of his treatment method, Schwartz reports an impressive 75 to 80 percent improvement in reducing the disabling symptoms of OCD.

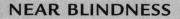

NEAR BLINDNESS

In the past, the most common conditions in the United States causing blindness were glaucoma, diabetic retinopathy, and macular degeneration. But, since there are now many effective treatments for glaucoma and laser treatments for diabetic retinal disease, these two diseases now cause blindness much less frequently. But, unfortunately, treatments for macular degeneration are usually much less effective. This insidious illness slowly damages the retina of the eye, causing blindness first in the center of the visual field and later, in some patients, spreading to block out almost their entire visual field.

Juliana is a delightful ninety-five-year-old, petite and perky, mentally sharp, a former classical ballet dancer and teacher. She suffers from severe macular degeneration and is nearly blind. Juliana also has poor hearing, peripheral neuropathy (chronic numbness and tingling in her feet), and high blood pressure. The only time I had to hospitalize Juliana occurred when she passed out unconscious in her church parking lot after a Sunday service. Her workup found that the likely cause of her brief unconsciousness was a transient drop in her blood pressure. Her treatment only necessitated lowering the dose of her blood pressure medication. I came to visit her early each morning in her hospital room. But, when I arrived, I would find Juliana was already up sitting in a chair, with a smile on her face, listening through headphones to her favorite classical music audiotapes. I remember thinking to myself that Juliana was benefiting from her own type of music meditation. Her blindness didn't at all interfere with her capacity to stimulate her mind this way and still be happy while stuck in a hospital room. Perhaps her capacity to reduce stress and enjoy living by participating in a life filled with dance and music has something to do with her remarkable longevity.

Research by neuroscientists (which will be discussed in greater detail in Chapter 7) has proven that when people lose their sight, they start to recruit areas of their brain that were formerly used to process visual information to process input from their senses of hearing and touch. This expands their ability to finely discern sound and tactile information.

This expanded hearing capability in people who are blind would make music meditation (page 134) particularly appealing for them. Also, Meditation on the Whole Person (page 119), which includes focusing awareness on sound, touch, taste, and smell, might be a very meaningful exercise.

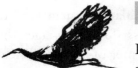

NEUROLOGICAL DISORDERS

In this category of illness, we will consider how meditation might benefit people who suffer from tension or migraine headache, stroke, mild cognitive impairment, or dementia from Alzheimer's disease.

TENSION AND MIGRAINE HEADACHE

Both tension and migraine headaches are precipitated, or made worse, by stress. I have seen several patients practice AH-OM Breath meditation (page 16) to relieve their stress, and also experience a big drop in the frequency of their headaches. Another tip to reduce tension headache is to maintain proper posture and alignment of the head and neck, especially when at work or reading. Stretching exercises and yoga can help with alignment and posture. Massage therapy and topical heat can reduce the headache and neck ache. For both tension and migraine headache prevention, getting enough sleep is important. (See the section in Chapter 4 "Meditations for a Good Night's Sleep" for detailed meditation instructions.)

For people with migraine headaches, it can be important to avoid certain food triggers like red wine, aged cheeses, foods with nitrates or sulfites, chocolate, and MSG. Women should pay attention to whether hormone changes associated with their menstrual cycle bring on migraines. (See prior section "Menopausal Symptoms and Premenstrual Syndrome" for a discussion of the usefulness of meditation with PMS.) In a society with a Starbuck's practically on every corner, trying to avoid excess caffeine intake can be a challenge, but doing so helps prevent caffeine withdrawal headaches, which are not uncommon.

STROKE

Stroke can produce a terrifying paralysis on one side of the body, sudden blindness, or an inability to speak. For the stroke victim and family members, this often results in a feeling of hopelessness and depression. Meditation can help overcome the sadness that occurs when a stroke victim constantly ruminates about the past, their loss of function, and what the future holds.

In his book *Still Here* (Riverhead Books, 2000), spiritual leader Ram Dass gives a fascinating account of his own experience of suddenly suffering a major stroke. This book is a wonderful account of how someone who has suffered a crippling stroke can use mindfulness to be a witness to their disability and still find meaning and happiness in life.

One medical study that shows meditation may be a way of lowering stroke risk was carried out by Dr. Amparo Castillo-Richmond's group and reported in the journal *Stroke* (2000). That study looked at the possible effect of meditation on the thickening of the walls of a person's carotid arteries (called IMT, which stands for intima-media thickness). Abnormal thickening of the carotid arteries, which supply much of the blood to the brain, is associated with increased risk of stroke. This randomized clinical trial studied 138 people, who also had hypertension, for up to nine months. Half of the test subjects engaged in health education classes, including home exercises twice daily. The rest of the test subjects practiced Transcendental Meditation (TM) for twenty minutes twice daily. The IMT for both groups was serially measured by a very accurate ultrasound device. During the study period, the TM group had a significant decrease in IMT by 0.098 mm, whereas the health-education control group had an average further thickening of IMT by 0.05 mm, for a difference of 0.15 mm between the two groups.

Exciting new information on stroke recovery is described in more detail in Chapter 7. It has now been determined that the brain has a previously unsuspected capacity to "rewire" itself to partially overcome brain damage caused by a stroke. And doctors are increasingly finding ways to speed up the rewiring of damaged brain tissue.

Trying to prevent another stroke by controlling blood pressure, high cholesterol, diabetes, and smoking cessation are other vital considerations in stroke patients.

MILD COGNITIVE IMPAIRMENT
AND ALZHEIMER'S DISEASE

There are varying degrees of cognitive impairment. Mild cognitive impairment (MCI) is a disorder that can progress to the more disabling condition of frank dementia known as Alzheimer's disease.

Mild Cognitive Impairment (MCI)

Mild cognitive impairment, a common disorder in the very elderly, is principally a problem of diminished short-term memory, often associated with mild problems in language or other mental function (such as ability to solve new problems). These difficulties are severe enough to be noticeable, but not severe enough to interfere seriously with daily life.

Some therapeutic strategies are now available to help prevent or reduce symptoms of MCI. Neuroscience research studies have shown that elderly people can preserve flexibility of mind and thinking ability (cognitive function) if they regularly engage in activities that are mentally challenging—but not so far beyond their abilities that they don't have a reasonable chance of success if they try hard. Activities such as socializing with other people and doing puzzles like sudoku and crossword puzzles, games like chess, bridge, and cribbage, and playing a musical instrument are possible examples. It also turns out that learning *new* skills later in life are a more effective means of slowing cognitive decline than just continuing to practice old previously acquired skills. Practicing meditation is another way older people reduce or prevent symptoms of MCI. Meditation preserves flexibility of mind by helping one to acquire new insights, rather than remaining stuck in old ways of viewing the world.

Neuroscientists have recently discovered that the brain of an older person is capable of producing new brain cells, and that physical exercise actually helps stimulate the formation of these new brain cells. This is likely why a recent study at Harvard found that walking just two or three hours per week improves memory and cognition in elderly people. Therefore, walking meditation should be an especially beneficial practice for elderly people who have MCI.

Alzheimer's Disease

Alzheimer's disease is a shocking and devastating progressive disorder of the brain that eventually renders people confused much of the time by robbing them of their memory, judgment, and problem-solving ability —and, in the end, even robs a person of much of their personality. More than 5 million people in the United States currently have been diagnosed with Alzheimer's disease, and the number is steadily rising with the "graying" of America. It is estimated that for people who live to be eighty-five years old, 50 percent will have Alzheimer's disease.

The inability of people with Alzheimer's disease to concentrate is one of the cardinal manifestations of the disease. This deficit makes it very difficult for people with this disease to meditate, except in the early stages of the disease. But, for someone who learned to meditate prior to the onset of Alzheimer's disease, practicing meditation like AH-OM Breath or relaxation response, as well as walking meditation, in the early stages of the disease *can* be very useful. This is because someone in the early stage of developing dementia symptoms is often well aware of their increasing difficulties of memory and declining overall function; and this usually causes them much frustration, fear, and anger. Meditation is potentially very beneficial to people with mild dementia, or MCI, because it can reduce these negative feelings and create more of a feeling of peaceful abiding and enjoyment in the wonderful things in life that are still available to them in the present.

Learning the practice of meditation can be quite beneficial to the family members (and other caregivers) who take care of people with Alzheimer's disease. Meditation can help them cope with the distress and fear of watching this unpredictable disease unfold in their loved one. For the family members, practicing mindfulness promotes an appreciation of the present moments of intimacy that can still be shared with their loved one before the dementia progresses to an advanced stage. Even in the later stages of Alzheimer's disease, when verbal communication is failing, a simple touch from a family member can nonverbally communicate love.

In the later stages of Alzheimer's disease, victims may be bedridden, incontinent of urine, and unable to recognize their family members; they may not even be able to talk. However, interestingly, when Alzheimer's or stroke patients can no longer talk, they often can still sing familiar songs. This is because, whereas language is mainly processed on the left side of the brain, music is processed on both sides of the brain. So, singing can be an important way of communicating with people who have dementia. I recall one of my patients, Sam, who lived to be 101 years old. In the last few years of his life, Sam had developed Alzheimer's disease and was eventually unable to speak any understandable words. But, when I went to visit him every month in the nursing home, I found that we could always connect on an emotional level by singing old familiar songs together. With clearly articulated words and melodic voice, Sam would sing songs like "On the Sunny Side of the Street," "The Band Played On," or his favorite song, "Happy Birthday."

For additional suggestions about how to minimize cognitive decline in aging individuals, including those with Alzheimer's disease, see the section in Chapter 7, "Learning and Wisdom."

OBESITY

Preventing obesity is important for good health. Weight control is also an important goal in the treatment and prevention of diabetes, which is becoming an epidemic in America. While diet fads come and go, the mainstay of treatment for obesity always comes back to decreasing the dietary intake of calories and increasing the amount of exercise, which burns off excess calories.

Weight lifting can help strengthen muscles but doesn't burn off calories efficiently. The type of exercise that is best for burning off calories is aerobic exercise, in which you work hard to move your leg and arm muscles repetitively for twenty minutes or more. For middle-aged and older people, the safest type of aerobic exercise is what is called low-impact aerobic exercise. This type of aerobic exercise minimizes the wear and tear on knee, hip, and ankle joints, which are vulnerable to degenerative arthritis and ligament and cartilage tears. Good examples of low-impact aerobic exercises are swimming, walking, and using a stationary bicycle, a stair-stepping machine, or elliptical exercise devices found at all fitness centers.

Walking meditation is a low-impact aerobic exercise, and can be the foundation of a healthy exercise program that helps control weight. Walking meditation also qualifies as a weight-bearing exercise that helps prevent osteoporosis. But you probably have to walk briskly for at least forty-five minutes to burn off a significant amount of calories. Meditation can also be practiced while doing more vigorous aerobic exercises, like riding a stationary bicycle or working out on an elliptical device, which burn off calories faster than walking.

On the caloric-intake side of the equation, there are a thousand different strategies for reducing food intake. A mostly vegetarian diet high in natural fiber is one diet strategy that seems to work well. Although, I confess that I have a hard time sticking to that diet consistently. For more details about the health benefits of a vegetarian diet, see Dr. T. Colin Campbell's book *The China Study: The Most Comprehensive Study of Nutrition Ever Conducted and the Startling Implications for Diet, Weight Loss and Long-term Health* (BenBella Books, 2006).

Some people become obese when they constantly snack on foods as a reaction to feelings of boredom or frustration. A meditation practice like AH-OM Breath, or the practices described in Chapter 4 called Buddha's Breathing Exercises or Meditation on the Whole Person, can transform and release these negative feelings. This would then help people avoid consuming large quantities of high-calorie "comfort foods," like ice cream and fried snack chips, as a way of dealing with difficult emotions. Also, during meditation, ideas for creative activities may come to mind, thus giving people stimulating things to do when they are not meditating, rather than just sitting around eating and watching television.

The meditation practice called Mindfulness of Eating can be a very effective way of reducing excess food intake. (To learn more about this practice, see Chapter 4, page 140.)

OSTEOARTHRITIS

Osteoarthritis is the most common form of arthritis. It is due to a degenerative process that wears down the joint cartilage and then the bone underneath. It can cause chronic pain in knees, hips, hands, back, or any joint. Unfortunately, there is no cure for this type of arthritis. But there are effective treatments to reduce symptoms.

The enormous numbers of people who have to cope with chronic arthritis pain make arthritis medications some of the biggest-selling medications. But these medications usually don't completely relieve all the pain. And some medications can have side effects like bleeding stomach ulcers, constipation, and liver and kidney damage. See the section "Meditations for Transforming Pain" in Chapter 4 to learn specific meditation techniques to reduce chronic pain. These meditation exercises can reduce chronic arthritis pain by 50 percent, making it far more tolerable.

If your osteoarthritis progresses to the point of requiring knee or hip surgery, meditation also can be useful in the postoperative recovery period. (See "Recovery from Surgery and Traumatic Injury," page 74.) And, in the physical therapy, rehabilitation phase of recovery from surgery, walking meditation can help heal the body, mind, and spirit all at the same time.

PAIN

Meditations to transform and reduce pain can be combined with physical treatments such as massage, physical therapy, chiropractic, or acupuncture. There is also nothing wrong with using appropriate doses of pain medication. But using these treatments in combination can minimize the use of *excess* pain medication, which is so often associated with side effects like constipation and nausea.

See Chapter 4, "Meditations for Transforming Pain" for detailed suggestions about how to use meditation techniques to diminish pain. There are many types of chronic pain syndromes that are amenable to this approach. These include conditions like osteoarthritis and cancer.

Postoperative surgical pain has been reduced by using guided meditation tapes or music therapy in the perioperative period, as discussed later in "Recovery from Surgery and Traumatic Injury" and "Music Meditation" and "Music Therapy" in Chapter 4.

A few examples of some other common painful conditions that respond to meditation are discussed next.

FIBROMYALGIA

Fibromyalgia is a poorly understood condition of unknown cause that manifests as chronic pain in many muscles of the back, neck, chest, arms, and thighs, often all at the same time. Ninety percent of people affected by this condition are women. Anti-inflammatory drugs, like ibuprofen, do little to help the condition since there is no significant degree of inflammation occurring to cause the pain. People who have this condition also have increased incidence of insomnia, irritable bowel syndrome, and/or depression.

Betsy is a forty-year-old woman with a long-standing history of fibromyalgia. Due to the pain, Betsy was unable to enjoy recreational activities or travel with her husband, and it was beginning to affect their marriage. I prescribed for Betsy a combination of sitting and walking meditation, massage therapy, yoga, and low-impact aerobic exercise. At times, I have also found that referral to a good acupuncturist or chiropractor can be very helpful in treating an acute flare-up of fibromyalgia. Betsy responded very well to these measures and returned to her normal activities. When she recently returned from a two-week trip with her husband to Thailand, she beamed with excitement when she told me how much she enjoyed visiting ancient temples and sightseeing.

Many women with fibromyalgia also suffer from depression. A randomized controlled trial by Sandra Sephton and colleagues, published in *Arthritis & Rheumatism* in 2007, studied ninety-one women with fibromyalgia who suffered from depression. Half the participants received the intervention of weekly classes in Mindfulness-Based Stress Reduction, compared to a control group that had no intervention. Depression was measured by standard tests. Depression scores at the beginning of the study were compared with depression scores after two months, and the intervention group improved significantly more than the control group. The study concluded that the "meditation-based intervention alleviated depressive symptoms among patients with fibromyalgia."

Another clinical trial studying fibromyalgia in seventy-seven patients was conducted by Kaplan and associates. In 1993, they published what they described as preliminary findings in the journal *General Hospital Psychiatry*. In that study (which had no control group), fibromyalgia patients learned (in weekly group classes) the meditation techniques of Mindfulness-Based Stress Reduction. At the end of ten weeks, 51 percent of the study patients showed moderate to marked improvement in measures like pain, fatigue, insomnia, and well-being. However, these results, showing a benefit from meditation in treating fibromyalgia, will be more convincing if they can later be confirmed in a large randomized controlled trial.

PAIN OF CHRONIC SHINGLES

Shingles is caused by infection with the varicella zoster virus, a virus in the herpes family that also causes chicken pox. Shingles usually first manifests as a localized, painful, blistering skin rash. The rash eventually subsides. But, in a few percentage of affected people, the virus does enough damage to the nerves under the surface of the skin to produce a burning, stinging, electric shock-like pain syndrome that can last for months or years, called post-herpetic neuralgia. There is a vaccine available to help prevent shingles. Unfortunately, about one-third of people vaccinated could still get shingles; however, they are less likely to get post-herpetic neuralgia.

I have had many patients with this unfortunate condition. But there is one such patient who always comes to mind. Rosemary is a highly educated woman in her fifties, who is married to a pharmaceutical chemist and has several grown children who are all "overachievers." She never had any serious health problem until she came down with shingles. Rosemary suffered for years afterward with an intense pain on the right side of her chest that never let up day or night. It drove her and her family crazy! By the time I saw her for the first time, she had already been to two cardiologists to be sure it wasn't heart trouble, an oncologist to be sure it wasn't cancer, a pulmonary doctor, a rheumatologist, an infectious disease specialist, and pain-management specialists, with no significant relief.

I was finally able to make Rosemary's pain much more bearable by recommending a combination of prescription medication, sitting meditation, and the meditation pain-control techniques described in Chapter 4. Once Rosemary found she was able to reassert some control over her pain, she became much less afraid of what the pain meant and was able to start focusing on enjoyable things in her life again. One of the most powerful techniques that worked for Rosemary was the modeling meditation exercise (page 132) in which she focused her awareness on the left side of her chest, the side that didn't hurt. Then she would try to model the movements of the painful right side of her chest after the normal left side, which markedly diminished the painful sensations.

PLANTAR FASCIITIS

Usually caused by repetitive traumatic injury, plantar fasciitis is a chronic painful tendonitis involving the big tendon that runs along the bottom of the foot. The injury often takes months to heal because of the daily need to walk on the injured foot. When I had to cope with the pain of plantar fasciitis for many months, neither anti-inflammatory drugs nor pain pills did much to reduce the pain. However, the same modeling meditation technique that Rosemary had used (mentioned above) also worked well for me. I eventually found that, rather than focusing on how much pain I felt in my injured foot, I could instead concentrate my awareness on how great it was that my good foot worked so well. I would then imagine that the painful foot was able to walk more like the good foot. Almost magically, the pain quickly became less intense and more tolerable. Months later, orthotic arch supports, stretching, temporarily avoiding reinjury from running or dancing, and time finally healed the injured tendon.

LOW BACK PAIN

Lisa, a beautiful young woman with long blond hair, is a licensed massage therapist. For many years she has had to cope with chronic low back pain due to her severe congenital scoliosis (abnormal curvature) of the spine. Unless you looked very closely, you wouldn't know she has this severely curved spine because Lisa has developed her muscles to hold her posture very straight. To help reduce her back pain, Lisa practiced the techniques described in Chapter 4 in the section "Meditations for Transforming Pain." Lisa would practice nonjudgmentally focusing her attention directly on her back pain. She would then imagine breathing in and out through an imaginary hole in the painful area of her back, and progressively relax her back muscles and reduce the pain with each out-breath. By using a combination of meditation, aerobic exercises, and yoga, Lisa was able to markedly reduce her chronic back pain. This enabled her to care for her one-year-old baby boy, take continuing education classes at a local college, and still work part-time as a massage therapist, despite her severe scoliosis.

Low back pain is an extremely common condition that causes suffering in many of my patients. Severe low back pain has many possible causes. Osteoarthritis is a common cause of back pain in elderly people. See the previous discussion of osteoarthritis. Also see the next section for a discussion of what to do when the facet joints of the back are not arthritic but just stuck together, which is called the facet syndrome.

One of the most common causes of low back pain in middle-aged people involves injuries to the intervertebral disks of the lumbar spine. In middle age, those disks (which normally act as shock absorbers for the spine) become more brittle. Then a surprisingly innocuous activity, like lifting groceries out of the car, or a bending motion of the back, like picking up a box or a small child, can cause microscopic tears to occur in the fibrous capsule of a disk. This injury causes inflammation and swelling of the disk, which then can put pressure on the nerves coming out of the spinal cord or pressure on the spinal cord itself. That can result in a severe jolt of pain in the back or down the leg from a simple awkward reaching movement, or from just getting up out of bed in the morning.

In this situation, in addition to meditations for pain control, it helps to take a mindful approach to proper alignment of the spine and balanced movements of the body. Also, be mindful of ordinary movements that you need to avoid, like awkward bending, twisting movements. Be aware that sitting for a long time in a straight-back chair puts a tremendous load on the lumbar spine. If you suffer from this condition, it is much better to sit in a recliner chair, where the weight of the back is distributed along the back of the chair, rather than sitting upright with all your weight resting on the injured disks. Intermittent use of a heating pad can also provide temporary relief. In over 95 percent of the cases, the body will eventually repair the disk injury and you can then return to more normal activities after giving your body a chance to heal. Meanwhile, mindful breathing and massage to ease the pain, attention to proper posture during daily activities, and meditation will help prevent the need for more radical treatments, such as back surgery.

Engaging in regular aerobic exercise—where the heart rate is elevated and you "break a sweat"—as well as practicing muscular strengthening exercises, like abdominal crunches and leg lifts, helps to support the back, restore function, and prevent reinjury.

Caution: If these suggestions don't work to help reduce your back pain, you should see a doctor for a more specific diagnosis and treatment recommendation, since there are many causes of back pain, some of which are due to a more serious underlying illness or injury.

MIDDLE BACK PAIN AND THE FACET SYNDROME

The most common cause of acute pain in the middle of the back is muscular strain, which will usually resolve in due course with proper rest, heat, and over-the-counter pain medication. The most common cause of chronic middle back pain is "the facet syndrome," which is also a frequent cause of low back pain. The vertebral bones of the back stack up, one on top of the other; and the facet joints are the contact points of the vertebral bones that actually support most of the weight. (The disks are the other critical weight-supporting structures.) When a person spends a lot of time sitting at home or at work, or driving long distances in a car, these facet joints become compacted and stuck in place. This results in a limited range of motion of the spine, and causes pain to emanate from tiny nerves in these facet joints. This is called the facet syndrome. One way to free up these stuck facet joints is to see a chiropractor or osteopathic doctor for spinal manipulation, which works very well. The problem is that the facet joints often rapidly become stuck together again, requiring frequent return visits to the chiropractor to "pop" them open again.

Meditations for transforming pain and the other techniques described in Chapter 4 can help relieve mid-back pain. In addition, I have found that self-treatment by stretching these stuck facet joints can be a very effective way to relieve recurrent mid-back pain quickly. These stretches can also be done several times a day to prevent mid-back pain. I approach doing these stretches in a mindful, unhurried fashion, almost like a meditation. I concentrate my entire attention on feeling the focal point of the stretch, while paying attention to my breath and the feeling of stretching the back muscles and popping open the facet joints. I position myself by lying down on the floor or in bed (to neutralize gravity) with my knees bent. Or I may sit back in a recliner chair or on a sofa with a firm, small pillow behind my back. I focus my weight directly on whatever area of my back is painful, stiff, or tight. I take a deep breath and hold it, and very slowly and gently rotate my back to the left while moving my right chest and shoulder slightly forward a couple of inches. The stretch is sustained until I feel the "pop" or "click" that occurs when the stuck facet joint releases and the range of motion of my back suddenly improves.

Depending on what part of the back seems locked or tight, I may try exhaling some of the air and repeating the same stretch maneuver. Doing that will stretch open the facet joints at a different level of the spine. In order to stretch the facet joints on the left side of the spine, I do the same twisting motion, rotating my back to the right, while slowly moving the left side of the chest and shoulder forward a couple of inches— *not* doing it in a ballistic or forceful way. I do a similar back stretch when I take my morning bath. I call it "bathtub chiropractic."

Another good stretch for the middle back is to lie down on your left side, hold your breath, and then stretch and curve your back upward. Maintain that stretch for a few seconds while moving the right side of your chest forward an inch. You might then feel a whole series of right-sided facet joints in the middle back "pop" open, releasing pain and stiffness there. Then, turn over onto your right side and do the same type of stretching technique to open up the mid-back facet joints on the left side.

Some yoga exercises can also quite effectively stretch the back and free up the facet joints. As noted before, you should see a doctor for an evaluation if these stretching techniques fail to relieve your back pain.

PREGNANCY

Pregnancy is, of course, not an illness. But it is a condition often associated with some challenging problems. When my wife, Jackie, gave birth to our first daughter, Shenandoah, she had to endure a terrible sixteen hours of labor. At the time, it seemed like it would never end. (Fortunately, our second daughter, Jasmine, came out so fast there was barely time for the obstetrician to get there and catch her as she came out.) Jackie used the Lamaze breathing technique to reduce the severe uterine contraction pains she had to endure. This mindful breathing technique is very similar to the heavy-breathing meditation exercise described earlier in Chapter 1.

Other problems pregnant women commonly encounter include low back pain, excess pregnancy weight gain, and depression (which can be quite severe in the weeks after giving birth). Drug therapy of pregnancy symptoms is fraught with risk of causing harm to the fetus as a side effect of giving medication to the mother. Many drugs are also excreted in breast milk, potentially harming a breast-feeding baby.

Therefore, using massage, topical heat, and the meditation techniques described on pages 130–133 for transforming pain are the safest ways to treat chronic pain in pregnancy. Taking advantage of the practice called Mindfulness of Eating and meditating on The Five Contemplations, described in Chapter 4, can help prevent excess pregnancy weight gain. The AH-OM Breath meditation practice can safely help prevent or treat pregnancy-associated depression. This calming meditation would also likely have a beneficial effect by allowing the fetus to grow and develop in a calm environment.

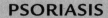

PSORIASIS

Psoriasis is a skin condition that causes a rash with large red, scaly plaques in many areas of the body at once. People with this condition may feel too embarrassed to swim in a public pool, since other people often incorrectly think the rash is contagious. Psoriasis can also cause systemic problems of gout and arthritis. Many cases of psoriasis skin rash can easily be controlled with topical creams. But some cases are much more severe, requiring multiple medications and phototherapy with ultraviolet light.

In 1998, Jon Kabat-Zinn's group at the University of Massachusetts Stress Reduction Clinic published in the journal *Psychosomatic Medicine* a randomized controlled trial of thirty-seven psoriasis patients who were undergoing phototherapy. They were randomized with one group listening to a guided mindfulness meditation audiotape while receiving light therapy, and a control group that just got the light therapy with no audiotape instructions. The results of post-treatment patient photographs were analyzed by doctors who were not told which patients used the meditation tapes (a single-blind study). The conclusion of the study was that the meditation group had a statistically significant increase in the rate of healing the psoriasis skin lesions.

RECOVERY FROM SURGERY AND TRAUMATIC INJURY

One study by the Blue Shield insurance company found that preoperatively providing a guided relaxation tape to surgery patients seemed to speed their recovery from surgery and reduce their length of stay in the hospital, saving Blue Shield an average of two thousand dollars per surgery. The patients who listened to the relaxation tapes also felt a greater sense of healing. A randomized trial of patients undergoing elective colorectal surgery was conducted by D. L. Tusek and his associates at the Cleveland Clinic, and reported in *Diseases of the Colon and Rectum*. They found that the group of patients who used guided-imagery tapes had less postoperative pain, anxiety, and morphine use than the control patients.

Ulf Nilsson and colleagues reported on a controlled clinical trial involving 151 patients studying the effect of music on postoperative surgical pain in the journal *Anesthesia*. That 2003 study demonstrated surgery patients treated with music-therapy tapes had less postoperative pain and required less morphine than the control group who didn't listen to music.

I compiled music-therapy CDs in eight different musical genres for Tri-City Medical Center in Oceanside, California. Surgery patients there have the option of listening to the music CDs in the preoperative and posterative surgery units. These music CDs have helped many patients cope with the fear and anxiety and postoperative pain from their surgery. They have helped other patients being treated on the medical floor cope with the anxiety and boredom of their hospital stay. When someone feels happy after listening to one of these CDs, it makes me happy too.

A randomized controlled trial conducted by Herbert Benson's group at Harvard Medical School studied twenty-seven patients after cardiac surgery, randomly assigned to two treatment groups. Both groups received standard postoperative medication therapies. The group that had been taught the meditation technique known as the Relaxation Response had a statistically significant decrease in a heart rhythm disturbance called supraventricular tachycardia, as well as greater decreases in psychological tension and anger, compared to the control group of patients, who just received educational information.

A possible explanation for meditation's capacity to reduce blood pressure, heart rate, and heart rhythm disturbances is, in part, a reduction in blood levels of adrenaline, the main hormone that mediates emotional arousal throughout your body. One prospective randomized study of heart failure patients by Curiati and colleagues did indeed find lower adrenaline blood levels in the patients who were taught to meditate.

Regardless of whether an injury results in fractures, sprains, lacerations, bruises, or the need for surgery, the meditation techniques for transforming pain can be used to reduce posttraumatic pain. Also, practicing the exercise called Meditation on the Whole Person can remind the injured person that they are far more than their injury, and can help restore their sense of well-being.

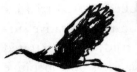

TERMINAL ILLNESS—DYING

If a dying person has been introduced to meditation before becoming gravely ill, he or she will be able to draw upon the energy of meditation to enhance well-being at the end of life. But, it is difficult for someone to learn a meditation practice in the final stages of a terminal illness, because one's energy level is low and the ability to concentrate may be limited. So it behooves us to work through these end-of-life issues when we are not gravely ill and still have the energy to concentrate on doing this work.

A dying person may not even have enough energy for conversation. But calm, peaceful abiding alongside the dying person, breathing with them, and gentle touching can communicate a lot nonverbally. Just deep listening, a few words of loving speech, or playing beautiful, familiar music can be very healing to the spirit of all people assembled. Recounting previous good times is a helpful focus for discussion when family and friends gather at the bedside of a dying loved one or at a memorial service. This activity can begin to help heal the painful loss.

The practice of meditation can help the surviving family members and friends to suffer less, making it easier for them to work through the bereavement process with a greater sense of acceptance and equanimity.

A hospice group in San Francisco called the Zen Hospice Project, founded by Frank Ostaseski, who is also the founder and current director of the Metta Institute (www.mettainstitute.org), is organized around the principles of Zen. Ostaseski has written that "the reflection on death is life affirming. When we come into contact with the precariousness of life, we also begin to appreciate how precious it is, and then we want to live more fully."

I have given workshop lectures on meditation to a group of hospice nurses and counselors who work at my local hospital and in the surrounding community. I know these hospice workers have used meditation to help themselves cope with their stressful compassionate work. They have also passed along some of these meditation concepts to patients and patients' family members.

In the next chapter, the section "Birth and Death" discusses a Zen-like perspective on death that can allow us to more easily accept it as a natural process of which we are all part. Practicing a meditation exercise called The Five Remembrances (page 123), which specifically focuses on the inevitability of illness and death, can help liberate us from obsessing about the fear of death.

A state of acceptance of death is exemplified by a unique statue of the Buddha that resides in the Wat Pho Buddhist Temple in Bangkok, Thailand. Instead of the usual sitting posture of most Buddha statues, this statue shows Buddha lying down when he was about to die, and depicts the moment he achieved Nirvana. At the time of dying, instead of fear and loathing, Buddha is seen (in the ultimate dimension) to be smiling, as he is about to enter Nirvana (see Figure 1 below).

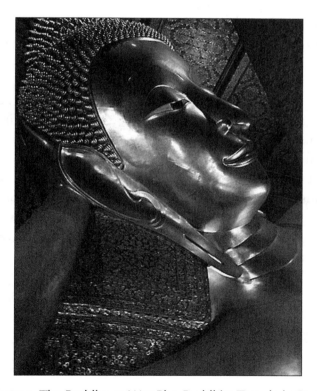

FIGURE 1. The Buddha at Wat Pho Buddhist Temple in Bangkok.

At the time of dying, instead of fear and loathing, Buddha is seen
(in the ultimate dimension) to be smiling, as he is about to enter Nirvana.

WHOLE-PERSON HEALTH CARE

The best medical care is practiced in such a way that the whole person's health and well-being—the elements of body, mind, and spirit—are all considered to be important. The doctor and patient ideally should form a partnership with shared responsibility for healthcare decisions, based on mutual respect and individual patient preferences. An approach to dealing with a health problem that works well for one patient may not be the best option for another patient. The qualities of compassion, loving-kindness, honest communication, and deep listening are ingredients in an optimal therapeutic partnership between a person and their doctor.

I want my patients to have the very best medications, high-tech devices, and diagnostic tools that modern medicine has to offer. Meditation is only one of a mix of treatments I might recommend. For some conditions, prescription medication or even surgery may be the best way to cure an illness.

For other conditions, alternatives to traditional medicine, called complementary therapies, can be beneficial as a part of the entire mosaic of healing. This might mean including one or more of the following types of complementary therapies: chiropractic, acupuncture, massage therapy, physical therapy, fitness training, stretching exercises, yoga, or nutritional counseling. A medical approach that combines, or integrates, traditional medicine with complementary treatments has lately been called "integrative health care." I like to practice integrative medicine, but I still like the term "whole-person health care."

CHAPTER THREE

Zen Perspective

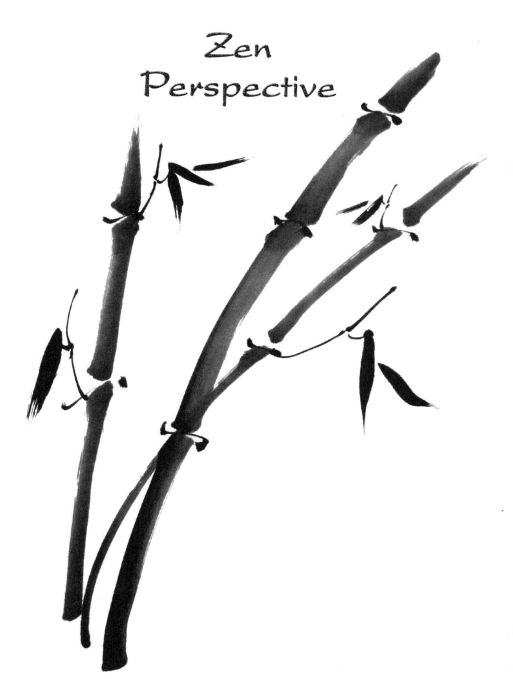

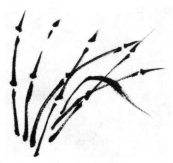

By now you have learned how to meditate. But how does meditation fit in with the other activities and challenges of your life? How can you avoid the fragmentation that comes from randomly jumping from activity to activity? How can you lead a balanced life that allows you to live your core principles every day?

The answer to these questions requires one to develop a coherent philosophy of life that is compatible with the laws of nature. This philosophy of life becomes part of the *spiritual* realm of your life. Bringing this spiritual dimension to your practice deepens your motivation to practice meditation regularly and sustains your commitment to the process. This gives you the determination to stick with it, through whatever difficulties you experience or no matter how busy or fragmented your life becomes. Meditation becomes a skillful way to link the spiritual to the physical dimension of your life.

In studying how various spiritual leaders have incorporated meditation into their lives, I find the insights of Zen Buddhism to be a very useful point of reference. While I don't subscribe to all aspects of Zen teaching, the concepts are truly enlightened and worth considering, especially because Zen speaks so directly to the healing power of meditation. I am not talking about Zen as a religion, but rather as a philosophy of life that is compatible with most religious beliefs and modern scientific theories. In the *Time* magazine cover story "The Dalai Lama's Journey" (March 31, 2008), reporter Pico Iyer explains that Buddhism is "more accurately called a science of mind than a religion."

Zen philosophy can deepen and enhance one's spirituality regardless of one's religion. And it's okay *not* to agree with all of the aspects of this perspective and still use what part of it works for you. The Zen perspective does not pretend to be the absolute truth, but invites you to explore life for yourself and draw your own conclusions, as there are many paths to spiritual enlightenment.

The fundamental aspects of the Zen perspective on life are outlined in this chapter. You will see how these concepts are incorporated into the other meditation exercises and practices described in Chapters 4 and 5.

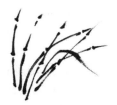

THE FOUR NOBLE TRUTHS

What evolved into Zen Buddhism began over 2,500 years ago in India as the teachings of an historical figure whose name was Siddhartha Gautama. He came to be called the Buddha, which in Sanskrit means "the Awakened One."

The core of Siddhartha Gautama's teachings starts with what he called the Four Noble Truths. These truths describe the existence of human suffering, the cause of human suffering, the ability to overcome suffering, and a path leading to the cessation of suffering.

FIRST NOBLE TRUTH

The first noble truth is that life contains suffering, called *dukkha* in Sanskrit. In other words, dukkha happens! Even people who seem to have charmed lives will eventually experience sickness, injuries, old age, and death. Siddhartha also taught, "Sadness, anger, jealousy, worry, anxiety, fear, and despair are suffering. Separation from loved ones is suffering. Association with those you hate is suffering. Desire, attachment, and clinging are suffering."

SECOND NOBLE TRUTH

The second noble truth is that all suffering is caused by overattachment to, or desire for, things that are impermanent. And, in fact, all things in the universe are impermanent and everything is in a constant state of change—even the things that seem so permanent. For example, while living in the Pacific Northwest in 1981, I witnessed what had appeared to be a massive, permanent mountain suddenly and radically change when a volcanic explosion blew the top off Mount St. Helens. Since moving back to Southern California, I have witnessed wildfires that swiftly consume people's homes and life-long possessions in the inferno of a summer firestorm. Another example of impermanence is demonstrated by global warming, which is causing profound changes in what had been centuries-old stable ecosystems. Even stars are impermanent.

The Hubble Space Telescope has captured images of distant older stars exploding in a supernova. Thus, we infer that even our own sun will eventually suffer a similar fate.

On the human level, we see that all people age and change. Right now many of the older cells in our own bodies are dying, while many other new cells are simultaneously being born. More than 2 million new red blood cells are born in your bone marrow each second! And your older red blood cells are dying at an equal rate. Like water spilling over a waterfall, our lives are an endless falling away of all experience. Pleasure, pain, loss, gain, fame, shame—it's all part of an endless passing show. The end of birth is death; the end of accumulation is dispersion; the end of meeting is separation. Everything arises, develops, and passes away. So we need to learn to live with the knowledge that nothing lasts forever.

THIRD NOBLE TRUTH

While the first two noble truths are pessimistic, the third is quite optimistic. The third truth says that the cessation of suffering is possible. Happiness and joy are possible in the here and now. You don't have to wait until after you die. It is possible to achieve a state of ultimate peace, understanding, happiness, and freedom called enlightenment.

FOURTH NOBLE TRUTH

The fourth noble truth is a description of a path that leads to enlightenment and the cessation of suffering. The pathway to enlightenment was described by Siddhartha as the Noble Eightfold Path of right understanding, right thought, right speech, right action, right livelihood, right effort, right mindfulness, and right concentration.

But, instead of describing the path as divided into eight separate elements, the path to enlightenment can be more simply summarized as the practice of a balanced combination of wisdom, morality, and meditation. I call these the three keys that open the door to enlightenment. What follows is a detailed description of the three keys to enlightenment.

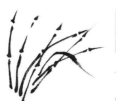

WISDOM: THE FIRST KEY TO ENLIGHTENMENT

Wisdom is also called insight, or *prajna* in Sanskrit. Wisdom includes insights gained from truly understanding the nature of impermanence, interconnectedness, nonattachment, and compassion. Wisdom may be attained by study, life experience (the school of hard knocks), or meditation.

UNDERSTAND IMPERMANENCE

Most people readily agree to the theory of impermanence, but they then proceed to live their lives as though things like their homes, loved ones, and institutions will always be there. By contrast, the Zen practice is to keep the insight of impermanence alive in every moment of daily life, and to always keep in mind that nothing is permanent.

However, don't think of impermanence as a pessimistic note in the song of life. It can actually be the very foundation of happiness, and can help you live deeply in every moment of your daily life. This is because when you realize that all things are impermanent, you begin to more deeply cherish what is wondrous in the here and now. You start to appreciate the ordinary, mundane things, like the building where you work, or the road upon which you drive, or the peaceful little community where you live, because you know those things won't always be there. You no longer see your loved ones moving through your life as in a dream. You want to look deeply into the eyes of your loved one and fully appreciate his or her presence in this very moment. Even difficult people become more tolerable, because you know the difficulties they pose are also impermanent.

REALIZE YOUR INTERCONNECTEDNESS

We can go beyond seeing ourselves as separate from the rest of the universe. We can come to realize that all things are interconnected and interdependent—that all things rely upon supports, both seen and unseen, for their existence. This is so, because that is so. (Or this is not so, because that is not so. Or this is so, because that is not so.) Modern-day Zen master Thich Nhat Hanh calls this "inter-being." I would qualify this idea by saying that all things are not equally interdependent. While a complex mosaic of connections is undeniable, there is a variable effect of one thing or person on another.

The wisdom of interconnectedness teaches us there is no separate self; and that we are only able to exist because of a multitude of enabling conditions. The wisdom of impermanence tells us there is no permanent self. Some Zen philosophers contend there is no self at all, saying that what seems like a self is just an aggregation of five constantly changing components: the body (form), feelings, perceptions, mental formations, and consciousness. I prefer to take a middle position and not deny what seems obvious: at some level *there is a self, but it is not a separate or a permanent self.* Buddha used the somewhat confusing phrase "emptiness of self" to mean that all things lack a permanent, separate self. But, this is just another way to refer to the impermanence and interconnectedness of all things.

CULTIVATE NONATTACHMENT

The wisdom of nonattachment teaches that you can reduce life's suffering by avoiding clinging to, or craving for, impermanent things like money, good food, sex, fame, power, and youth. Reducing your attachment to these impermanent things increases your sense of freedom. Also you can practice nonattachment by letting go of negative thoughts and feelings that will in the end diminish your happiness, such as grudges, jealousies, hatred, fears, and intolerance.

Don't be so attached to the drama of your life. This will enable you to minimize the negative emotions that disappointments bring. Learn to be a witness to your life as it unfolds, without dwelling in judgment, regrets, or angst.

Avoid attachment to the notion of a permanent, separate self. This includes accepting the knowledge that your own life is impermanent and that your death is inevitable. The insight of "no separate self" also helps you avoid selfish attachments and arrogance. Too little self-esteem can be a source of unhappiness, but too much self-esteem and lack of humility is also a negative trait. The following prayer I heard at Deer Park Monastery offers an interesting perspective on the relationship between the self and other people: "Deliver us from the inferiority complex. Deliver us from the superiority complex. And also deliver us from the equality complex." Reciting this prayer helps to diminish the illusion of a permanent, separate self; but the last line of the prayer also acknowledges that we are, each of us, a unique self.

It is also important to understand that the practice of nonattachment doesn't mean *no* attachment. Even Buddhist monks and nuns, who are less attached to external things than are lay people, form attachments to their fellow monastics and teachers. Lay practitioners often have healthy attachments to things like their family and their job. It is okay to form some degree of nourishing attachments in our lives; but the key is to avoid overattachment, clinging, and the inability to let go.

When considering our attachments, it is interesting to look at some old photographs that were taken during some of the best times of our lives. When I look at a bunch of these old photos, I am struck by how amazing our lives are. And, viewed through the prism of time, I see that these past good times were actually quite fleeting and impermanent. I sometimes wonder was that person in the old photos really me? He looks similar. But I know that most of the cells that were alive in me years ago have long since died, to be replaced by new cells. The memories seem to provide a type of continuity, but the person that is me has totally transformed.

Indeed, if we and our lives are like a constantly changing river, is there anything that can truly be grasped or clung to? So, when you hold your loved ones in your arms, don't try to grasp them too tightly, because it is an illusion that they are there for you in a permanent way. They, like you, are a constantly changing flow. One cannot grasp a constantly changing flow. It will just slip through your fingers. So appreciate your life and your loved ones without grasping or clinging too tightly to the illusion that you can ever hold on to them permanently.

Our attachments, which are based on love and compassion for other people, may indeed lead to some suffering. But that's okay. Buddha distinguished between different types of suffering. He concluded that this type of suffering, which can motivate right action and acts of loving-kindness toward other people, is acceptable. And this type of suffering is far less severe than the suffering that occurs as a consequence of clinging to and craving sensory pleasures.

PRACTICE COMPASSION

Compassion (*karuna* in Sanskrit) is the desire to help reduce the suffering of others. The Dalai Lama, a Tibetan Buddhist, has said, "If you want others to be happy, practice compassion. If you want to be happy, practice compassion." This is because, as we will discuss in Chapter 7, our brains are hardwired to feel compassion for other people. Additionally, the knowledge of impermanence leads us to a sympathetic feeling of compassion for other people (as well as for animals, plants, and minerals), because, like us, they too are impermanent and eventually experience suffering and loss. Awareness of interconnectedness means we should extend our feelings of compassion even to people we view as enemies. This is because those unpleasant people are closely connected to us as part of the fabric of our wondrous lives, and their negative behaviors can also help us to see our own flaws.

All humans suffer. But you can make use of that suffering. You can learn from it, and it can nourish your understanding and compassion. Don't fear that if you have too much compassion, you will lose yourself. Learning to listen with compassion will help prevent you from suffering from other people's angry or unkind words and actions. This is because you will understand that someone's unkind behavior is often born of their own suffering. And you will understand that everything is impermanent, even negative behavior. So protect yourself with compassion.

Love is the ultimate form of compassion. (There will be much more on the subject of love later in Chapter 5.) Compassion leads us to treat people with acts of loving-kindness and words of loving speech. Psychologist Marshall Rosenberg writes very well about how to learn to use loving speech. Dr. Rosenberg calls this type of speech "nonviolent communication." His book *Nonviolent Communication: A Language of Life* (PuddleDancer Press, 2003) elaborates on how to develop the skills to effectively communicate with others in a kind and compassionate way. This type of communication requires "deep listening," which means you attentively and sympathetically just listen to a suffering person tell you their story without interrupting them. This type of listening, all by itself, can help relieve a lot of suffering in the other person. An enlightened Zen practitioner, motivated by compassion to reduce the suffering of others and help guide them to enlightenment, is called a *bodhisattva*.

Also, have compassion for yourself. Forgive yourself for not being a perfect listener, a perfect spouse, a perfect practitioner. Nobody is perfect. In *Creating True Peace* (Free Press, 2003), Thich Nhat Hanh writes,

> The process of transformation and healing takes ongoing practice. We produce garbage every day, so we need to practice continuously to take care of our garbage in order to make it into flowers. There may be friends around us who seem to practice better than we do, but it is important to accept who we are and not reject ourselves or our efforts. If we have within us only 10 percent flowers and 90 percent garbage, we may wish we had 90 percent flowers and only 10 percent garbage, but this kind of thinking does not help. We have to accept the 90 percent garbage in us in order to be able to increase the 10 percent flowers to 12 percent, then 14 percent, then 20 percent. This acceptance will bring us peace and we will not be caught in an inner struggle. Even those who produce many flowers daily have garbage and must practice continuously. It is okay for us to have the mud of suffering if we know how to practice.

To summarize the foregoing, a Zen-like approach to life emphasizes the wisdom of looking deeply into the nature of impermanence and interconnectedness, and avoiding an overattachment to sensory pleasures. Compassion and kindness are encouraged, as well as living in harmony with other people.

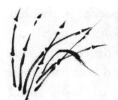

MORALITY: THE SECOND KEY TO ENLIGHTENMENT

Most of the moral principles of Zen Buddhism are succinctly described below in the section "Follow the Five Precepts." They are quite similar to codes of morality contained in most of the world's great humanistic and religious traditions. One moral principle that Buddhism emphasizes more than most other traditions is the value of being happy.

LIVE YOUR PRINCIPLES

In *A Path with Heart* (Bantam Books, 1993), psychologist and former Buddhist monk Jack Kornfield writes, "How can I live my spiritual practice, how can I bring it to flower in every day of my life?" Clarifying your core moral principles, developing your "moral compass," and consistently living a moral life may not always be easy. But employing skillful means to live your principles every day will contribute greatly to your ultimate peace and happiness.

FOLLOW THE FIVE PRECEPTS

As in all traditions, follow the golden rule of do unto others as you would have others do unto you. More specifically, in Zen Buddhism the Five Precepts are described as follows: refrain from killing, stealing, sexual misconduct, lying or harsh speech (instead practice loving speech and deep listening), and consumption of intoxicants (including avoiding toxic media such as movies, television shows, music, and books that glorify or sensationalize violence and other unhealthy behaviors).

BE HAPPY

Happiness is a centrally important Buddhist moral principle. Buddha taught that the pursuit of happiness is a moral imperative. *The Art of Happiness* (Simon & Schuster, 1998), a beautifully written book by the

Dalai Lama, begins this way: "I believe that the very purpose of our life is to seek happiness."

Thomas Jefferson, one of the "founding fathers" of the United States of America, wrote that same moral principle into the Declaration of Independence, which begins with the statement that people are entitled to "life, liberty, and the pursuit of happiness."

Happiness is not just a moral principle and a pleasant state of being. Practices that sustain happiness also have a direct positive impact on our health and longevity, as seen in the previous chapter's review of medical research literature on the health benefits of being happy.

So, self-serving as it may sound, seeking happiness is morally good. But what type of happiness? Zen teaches that we enhance our happiness when we promote positive mental states such as kindness, compassion, love, humility, generosity, and patience, and reduce the negative mental states of greed, jealousy, anger, hatred, arrogance, and intolerance.

The Dalai Lama has written that one of the best ways to increase happiness is this: "If you can, serve other people. If not, at least avoid harming them."

In a similar fashion, Buddha said, "Sympathetic joy arises when one rejoices over the happiness of others and wishes others well-being and success."

In *Old Path White Clouds: Walking in the Footsteps of the Buddha* (Parallax Press, 1991), Thich Nhat Hanh further elaborates on the Buddha's definition of happiness:

> "Happiness," Buddha said, "is not the result of gratifying sense pleasures. Sense pleasures give the illusion of happiness, but in fact they are sources of suffering . . . True happiness is living in ease and freedom, without clinging or aversion. A happy person cherishes the wonders taking place in the present moment—a cool breeze, the morning sky, a golden flower, a look filled with understanding, a loving word, a meal shared in warmth and awareness, the smile of a child. A happy person can appreciate these things without being bound by them. Understanding all dharmas are impermanent and without a separate self, a happy person does not become consumed even by such pleasures. Because he understands a flower will soon wilt, he is not sad when it does."

MEDITATION: THE THIRD KEY TO ENLIGHTENMENT

The Sanskrit word for meditation is *dhyana*. In Japanese, the word for sitting meditation is *zazen*. Regardless of the specific name used, meditation is the skillful means by which you can reduce physical and emotional suffering and increase peace and happiness.

THE FRUITS OF MEDITATION

The benefits of meditation are called the "fruits of the practice." The fruit of meditation is its capacity to diminish stress, fear, anger, arrogance, drowsiness, frustration, loneliness, and despair, as well as help heal health problems like high blood pressure and symptoms of chronic pain, psoriasis, premenstrual syndrome, tension headaches, fatigue, and a host of other physical ailments as described in Chapter 2. The other fruit of meditation is its capacity to increase happiness, energy, creativity, compassion, kindness, generosity, tolerance, insight, and peace.

THREE APPROACHES

Zen teachings contain three basic approaches to meditation. All three types of meditation are useful for a complete pathway to enlightenment. The first, most fundamental type is calming meditation. The AH-OM Breath meditation you have been practicing is a form of calming meditation. The second meditation technique is the acquisition of meditative insight. This form of meditation can help one gain insight into the root cause of suffering and/or transform negative states of mind. The third approach to meditation, called mindfulness, is practiced while doing normal daily activities.

A single meditation exercise may contain elements of all three types of meditation. Take, for example, walking meditation (page 105). This practice usually eases stress and quiets the mind. Therefore, it is a type of calming meditation. Walking meditation is also simply mindfulness of walking. Hence, it is a type of mindfulness practice. However, if you practice walking meditation while reciting a spiritual poem or phrase, it can help generate insight and becomes a type of insight meditation.

Calming Meditation

Calming meditation is like what was described by Ram Dass in *Be Here Now* (Hanuman Foundation, 1971) when he wrote, "Create in yourself an absolutely calm center where it is always right here and now. It is just light. It is just is-ness." Calming meditation relaxes the body and promotes positive mental states such as happiness, peace, and compassion. Besides AH-OM Breath, other examples of calming meditation are described in Chapter 4: Well-Being; Pebble Meditation; The Stress Reliever; Yoga Complete Breath; and music meditation. Body scan and other techniques of Mindfulness-Based Stress Reduction, which were both mentioned in the Chapter 2 discussion of stress, as well as Total Relaxation as practiced in the tradition of Thich Nhat Hanh, are all calming meditation methods.

Meditative Insight

Here we are talking about the capacity of meditation to produce insight. (This is not to be confused with the particular school of meditation called Insight Meditation, or Vipassana Meditation, which is an offshoot of Theravada Buddhism.)

Meditation produces insights that can enable one to transform negative mental states such as anger, jealousy, greed, chronic pain, intolerance, hate, and impatience. Previously cultivating the wisdom of impermanence, interconnectedness, nonattachment, and compassion can help one, during meditation, to attain insight into the root causes of one's suffering and how to reduce it.

As explained earlier, once the mind becomes very still, any form of meditation can be associated with spontaneous insight. You can also promote insight by meditatively repeating certain guidewords, a key phrase, chant, or *gatha* (Sanskrit for a spiritual poem). I will discuss much more about how to practice techniques that help generate insight in

Chapter 4, such as Buddha's Breathing Exercises, Meditation on the Whole Person, and meditations for transforming anger.

Mindfulness Is Meditation

Mindfulness is a type of meditation that can be practiced during normal daily activities. Mindfulness is the practice of concentrating your full attention on what you are currently doing or experiencing from moment to moment. Don't worry about the future or ruminate about the past; you simply dwell in the present, and witness what is happening without being critical or judgmental. However, this doesn't mean you are passive. On the contrary, you are much more alert and alive to what is happening right now. This practice may generate a sense of awe at the miracle of life, and you often feel more connected to your surroundings. If you train yourself to be mindful during ordinary daily activities, this will also enable you to reach deeper states of meditation during formal sitting meditation.

Ram Dass, in *Be Here Now,* describes a mindful approach to life this way: "When there is a task to do, you *are* the task." With mindfulness, the activity itself becomes the focus of your meditation, thus quieting the thinking mind and keeping you grounded in a present awareness. Mindfulness is practiced during ordinary activities of daily living, such as walking, eating, bathing, breathing, stretching, cleaning up the yard, holding hands, having sex, and while performing other simple activities.

Mindfulness of daily activities should not be confused with the formal sitting meditation method called mindfulness meditation. People who practice mindfulness meditation often sit in meditation for a defined period of time, such as ten to twenty minutes twice daily. The focal point of this meditation method is not just one thing, but *everything* that comes into the person's awareness—including feelings, thoughts, sounds, visual perceptions, and so on. All of it is regarded in a nonjudgmental way, and it all is given space to just be. When sitting in mindfulness meditation, one simply pays attention as an observer to whatever is there, without thinking about it. When the mind becomes still enough, insights about the roots of major problems can spring into consciousness.

On the other hand, the general term "mindfulness" refers to the practice of staying rooted in the present while doing everyday activities. When practicing mindfulness, don't allow yourself to get caught up in multitasking, trying to get several things done at once. When you are mindful there should be *no hurry*. Hurrying to get something done is thinking about the future; whereas mindfulness, like all meditation, is peacefully abiding in the present. Thich Nhat Hanh describes this "no hurry" state of being as like the feeling of "I have arrived. I am home in the here, in the now."

There are some important activities and responsibilities in everyone's life that requires thinking. So, one usually does not practice mindfulness *all* day long. But, when you are doing simple daily activities, don't let the thinking mind dominate your awareness. It's okay to notice thoughts as they occur, but don't stay attached to them. Simply, and noncritically, note any thoughts, and then gently redirect your mind back to your breath and the activity at hand. Focusing attention on your breath for just three in-breaths and out-breaths quickly takes your awareness out of your head and reconnects your mind to what's going on in your body. Try to avoid naming or labeling things you see or hear, because naming things inevitably triggers a thought process. The thinking mind then becomes quiet, like the calm stillness in a reflecting pool of water.

As another example of how this works, let's say you are about to drink a glass of iced pink lemonade. Don't grab the glass on the run and gulp it down—while, at the same time, you are thinking about where you are going and what will happen when you get there. Instead, be mindful, slow down, and focus your entire attention on the act of drinking the lemonade. You might notice how wonderful it is that all you have to do is to will your arm and hand to reach for the pitcher of lemonade, and your arm and hand automatically pick up the pitcher and accurately pour just the right amount of the liquid into a glass without spilling it. That, in itself, is a minor miracle. You raise the glass to your lips in a beautifully coordinated fashion. You smell the fresh aroma of the lemon, see the pleasing pink color of the liquid, and feel the refreshing taste of the lemonade, so fruity and slightly tangy as it bathes your tongue. You feel the cool, hard contours of the ice and the softer texture of the lemon pulp. You feel thirst-quenching satisfaction as you easily swallow it down, without aspiring any into your windpipe—another miracle of coordination. You don't have to think about it, or express it in words, as I just did. You simply experience it fully—moment to moment. Without trying, that satisfying act of mindful drinking will help reduce your stress and gladden your mind.

It takes practice to learn to spend more of your time in this mindfulness state. But don't worry that you don't get it right all the time. You can just relax and not hurry because you have already arrived. With mindfulness, you become more fully aware of who you truly are right now. Zen teaching is full of thought puzzles called koans. One of these paradoxical puzzles teaches that the goal of Zen is "to arrive at the beginning." We learn these techniques and practices in order to awaken to what our true nature was like when we had the childlike wonder of a beginner's mind.

ENLIGHTENMENT

Enlightenment is the state of ultimate peace, understanding, happiness, and freedom. In other languages, enlightenment goes by different names. It is called *satori* in Japanese, *wu* in Chinese, *Nirvana* in Sanskrit (the classical language of ancient India), and *nibbana* in Pali (the popular language of India in Buddha's time).

For most people, the path to enlightenment requires much practice to make substantial progress. But, the Zen school of Buddhism teaches it is possible for some people to achieve enlightenment through meditation by an almost mystical, direct intuitive insight, without the need for a logical understanding of Zen theory. In *Zen Buddhism: Selected Writings of D. T. Suzuki* (Three Leaves Press, 1956), Daisetz Suzuki, the Japanese scholar whose writings are one of the first authoritative accounts of Zen published in the Western world, writes, "Sartori may be defined as an intuitive looking into the nature of things in contradistinction to the analytical or logical understanding of it."

However, for most of us, the path to enlightenment takes a dedicated application of the skillful means described in this chapter. While there are many aspects to these skillful means, in *Old Path White Clouds,* Thich Nhat Hanh simplifies the essence of the path poetically this way: "Look at all things with awareness, take peaceful steps, and smile with compassion."

Just as there are many paths to meditation, there is also no one best path to enlightenment. The Buddha described what he called "right view," which includes the assertion that *no view is the absolute truth,* including the Zen Buddhist view. Keeping this insight in mind prevents us being caught in a dogmatic, fundamentalist position and allows us to listen to other people's views with an open mind. Indeed, Nirvana is sometimes described as the absence of all views.

The wisdom contained in the Dharma can point one in the right direction along the path of more happiness and less suffering. However, Buddha admonished his followers not to cling to his, or any other, description of the way the universe works. He said, "The teaching is merely a vehicle to describe the truth. Don't mistake it for the truth itself. A finger pointing at the moon is not the moon itself. The finger is needed to know where to look for the moon, but if you mistake the finger for the moon, you will never know the real moon."

Another metaphor used by Buddha, as reported by Thich Nhat Hanh in *Old Path White Clouds,* is: "The teaching is like a raft that carries you to the other shore. The raft is needed, but is not the other shore . . . Use the raft to cross to the other shore, but don't hang on to it as your property. Do not become caught in the teaching. You must be able to let it go."

BIRTH AND DEATH

Whether or not we are aware of it, our views about birth and death have a large influence on our thoughts and actions in day-to-day life. By and large, the Zen perspective is compatible with most world religions. But, when it comes to concepts about birth and death, both Zen and science-based theories may contradict some religious views about God, the soul, and life after death. However, it's okay for someone to believe in those traditional religious views. As was just pointed out, Buddha taught that no view is the absolute truth, not even the Dharma. My own views are derived from an understanding of the available evidence and from personal experience, which is always limited at best. Also, a person may disagree with Zen concepts about birth and death and still benefit from applying the rest of the Zen perspective and the healing power of the meditation exercises to their life.

BIRTH IS NOT THE BEGINNING

Regarding our birth, we are not created from nothing. As previously stated, Zen takes a scientific-like view of causation. Things and thoughts are not created from nothing; they come about, or manifest, as a result of certain preceding conditions. This is so, because that is so. Prior to birth, a unique individual comes into being after the sperm from the father joins together with an egg from the mother. And the parent's genetic material is the manifestation of the union of preceding ancestors from endless generations past, like so many tributaries feeding into an endlessly flowing river.

Buddha also taught, "All beings, organic and inorganic, rely on the law of dependent co-arising. The source of one thing is all things."

In *Old Path White Clouds,* Thich Nhat Hanh goes on to explain, "The teaching on dependent co-arising . . . could be considered the heart of the Way of Awakening." Buddha said, "Things do not need a creator . . . they arise from one another . . . the one creates the many, and the many the one. If we look deeply, we can see the one in the many and the many in the one."

Buddha explained that when we look deeply into any person or object, we see it is the manifestation of a multitude of enabling conditions. Looked at from this perspective, a simple clay bowl, for example, has elements of clouds, rain, water, heat, sun, earth, air, human work, time, space, and so on, so that practically the entire universe has contributed to the manifestation of the bowl. The same applies to the manifestation of a person. Therefore, we don't come from nothing, and we don't come from just one source: "The source of one thing is all things."

CONTINUATION AFTER DEATH

After death, we don't become nothing. Physicist Albert Einstein first described the relationship between energy and matter as $E = MC^2$. This scientific equation states that a small amount of matter can potentially be converted into a very large amount of energy. Stated another way, matter is equivalent to very concentrated energy. Thus, our bodies are composed of very concentrated and highly organized energy. When a person dies, they don't become nothing. Their matter and energy are transformed but still remain in the universe. This is an expression of the scientific principle of the first law of thermodynamics, also called the conservation of energy.

Experiments in quantum physics (a branch of science that studies the behavior of matter and energy at its smallest—quantum—level) have demonstrated that energy waves (like light waves) can also act like particles. Other experiments have shown that particles, such as protons and electrons, can have wave-like properties. Therefore, it is possible to imagine that, on one level, our bodies are very concentrated energy waves moving through life, much like a wave moves through the ocean.

Zen teachers often compare our inevitable death to a wave crashing on the beach. After a wave crashes, the energy and water molecules still remain. Likewise, after our death our matter and energy will still remain in the universe but will have been transformed and eventually organized into different relationships. Thus, the energy and matter that is us will continue in some form after death. Siddhartha Gautama put it this way: "The temporal body arises from the four elements which dissolve only to endlessly recombine again." These elements will later recombine in new and previously unforeseen ways. No form is permanent.

Some Zen teachers have used another interesting metaphor for the continuity of birth and death. It has been said that our life is like a droplet of water cascading over a waterfall. While we are on the way down, we seem separate from the other drops of water. We shine and gleam in the sunlight in a variety of refracted and reflected colors. When the water droplets hit the bottom of the falls, they don't cease to exist. Most of the water droplets reform again into a flowing river, similar to the existence they had before they separated temporarily at the top of the waterfall. Similarly, after death our matter and energy don't cease to exist. Instead, they continue in other forms.

Another very important form of our continuation is the enduring effects of our previous words and actions. We are also "continued" by our children, grandchildren, great-grandchildren, and beyond.

Many Zen masters teach that, because of these various forms of continuation, there is no such thing as death. But, it seems clear to me that after death fundamental and irreversible change does occur. The highly organized matter and energy that is our body permanently dissipates, part of which may later reform into other organized groupings. It also seems clear that there will be no further words or actions from the deceased person. However, as another part of our continuation, there likely will be unforeseen future effects of our past words, thoughts, actions, and quality of being. Part of our essence thus lives on in the hearts and minds of people that have been, or will be, touched by our previous words and deeds.

NO PERMANENT SOUL

Thich Nhat Hanh teaches that the law of impermanence also applies to the understanding that there is no permanent soul. There is no soul that remains intact throughout time to transcend death and float off into the sky or to later inhabit another body. There *is* a soulful or spiritual dimension to our lives, but it is not as a permanent soul. Nothing is permanent.

WHEN DEATH APPROACHES

Viewed from this perspective, the death of a loved one is a sad event for the family and friends who survive. However, it makes sense that aging life forms must die in order to make room on this evolving planet earth for new forms to continually come into being. The classic Buddhist analogy is that the beautiful flower must die to become the compost that enables new, fresher flowers to later manifest. An understanding of this natural order, and knowing that people do continue in several ways after death, can help us to more easily accept the death of a loved one. Also, as discussed in Chapter 2, "Terminal Illness," meditation can comfort the survivors so they suffer less.

All things arise, develop, and pass away. Understanding impermanence, and knowing that after death our matter and energy remain in many forms as our continuation, helps us to accept the knowledge of our own eventual death. Coming to terms with the inevitability of your own death prevents you from clinging too much to the fear of losing your life. This will help liberate you and set you free.

A BRIEF HISTORY OF ZEN

The origin and evolution of Zen are very interesting. Siddhartha Gautama was born more than 2,500 years ago in 560 B.C.E. His parents were king and queen of the Northern Indian kingdom called Shakya (or Sakya), located at the foothills of the Himalayan Mountains in what is now Nepal. Siddhartha grew up as a prince, led a relatively comfortable early life, and received a good education.

During that same period in India many smaller kingdoms were becoming consolidated into larger kingdoms and cities, and new philosophical and religious ideas began to proliferate. The age-old tradition of Hindu Yoga meditation was well-known and practiced by local ascetic monks of the time. And there is even written evidence of meditation practices in India that date back more than 3,500 years.

At the age of twenty-nine, Siddhartha left the comforts of the palace where he had been raised, gave up nearly all of his possessions, and became an ascetic monk. Some of the practice methods he adopted, like meditation, were practices borrowed from other spiritual teachers and writings of which Siddhartha was well aware. Eventually, he became the great spiritual teacher known as the Buddha, or "the awakened one." He developed many of his insights about a path leading to enlightenment while practicing meditation. And he spent much of the rest of his life teaching others about his spiritual ideas and practices. Siddhartha is sometimes referred to as Shakyamuni Buddha (great sage of the Shakya clan), or the Tathagata, or Monk Gautama. (It helps to be acquainted with some of these names and other Sanskrit words in order to more easily read other books about Buddhism.) An excellent depiction of the life of the Buddha can be found in Thich Nhat Hanh's book *Old Path White Clouds.*

Siddhartha Gautama's teachings and their further elaboration are often collectively referred to as "the Dharma." After the death of Siddhartha at age eighty, his teachings spread throughout India and Sri Lanka (formerly called Ceylon), then to Tibet, China, Japan, Mongolia, Korea, and the Southeast Asian countries of Vietnam, Thailand, Cambodia, Laos, and Myanmar (Burma), as well as more recently to Europe, Australia, and North America. There developed two main branches of Buddhism: Theravada (which predominated in Sri Lanka and Southeast Asia) and Mahayana (which predominated in the northern Asian countries). And over the centuries, many different schools of Buddhism have developed as offshoots from these two main branches. Different schools placed more or less emphasis on various aspects of the Buddha's teaching.

Mahayana Buddhism was introduced in China in the second century. Chinese Buddhism began to blend with other local schools of thought, specifically Taoism (which emphasized a person's relationship to nature) and Confucianism (which dealt more with a person's relationship to other people). This Chinese version of Buddhism was called Ch'an. Ch'an Buddhism later spread to Japan where it came to be called Zen Buddhism, or simply Zen. One of the distinguishing characteristics of Zen is a very strong emphasis on the practice of meditation.

At the same time that the Ch'an and Zen schools of Buddhism were on the rise, many other schools of Buddhism continued to flourish. Some examples include Vajrayana (also called Tibetan Buddhism), Pure Land Buddhism, and Vipassana. To make it even more confusing, different Buddhist schools splintered into various sects. For example, there are six different sects of Tibetan Buddhism and even more offshoots of Zen. One of the most influential Chinese teachers of Ch'an (Zen) was Lin Chi (also called Rinzai in Japan), who lived in ninth-century China. Contemporary Zen master Thich Nhat Hanh, who is often referred to in this book, traces his Zen lineage directly back to the teachings of Lin Chi, which were brought to Vietnam by Chinese monks.

The ideas of Buddhism arrived much later to influence the Western cultures of Europe and North America. In the nineteenth century, American philosophers Henry David Thoreau (1817–1862) and Ralph Waldo Emerson (1803–1882) were aware of Buddhist teachings, which influenced the development of their philosophy of transcendentalism. In the nineteenth and twentieth centuries, many immigrants from Asian countries brought with them the practices of Buddhism. In the early twentieth century, German novelist Hermann Hesse incorporated ideas from Buddhism into his books *Siddhartha* (1922) and *Journey to the East* (1932). Later, the pop countercultural revolution of the late 1960s and 1970s was associated with increased interest in Buddhism and meditation in North America, parts of Europe, and Australia.

Current estimates of the number of Buddhists worldwide vary from 350 to 500 million. Today, almost all the schools of Buddhism are represented in North America. The majority of Buddhists practicing in the world today are not of the Zen school. However, all schools of Buddhism have much in common. That is why, for example, many of the writings of the Dalai Lama, a Tibetan Buddhist, bear a lot of similarities to the themes and conclusions found in Zen writings.

CHAPTER FOUR

Meditation and Healing Exercises for Expanding Your Practice

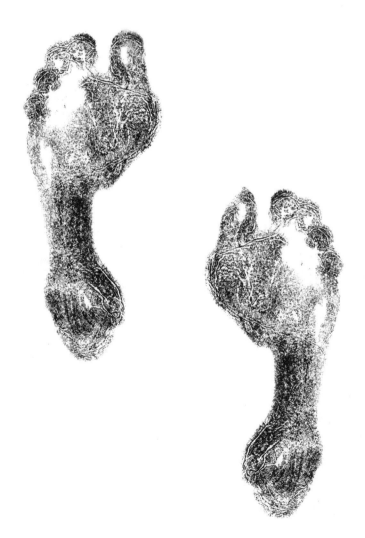

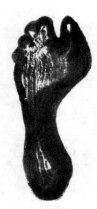

This chapter describes a series of traditional and contemporary meditations and practices. Included are calming meditations, as well as practices to promote meditative insight and mindfulness. These exercises will help expand your practice so you can benefit more from meditation's healing power.

Please do not attempt to make a regular practice of *all* of these techniques. Feel free to try either all or just some of these exercises, and use only the ones that seem to work best for you. You can choose to practice different meditation methods at different times. This choice of practice method may depend on factors such as your mood or temperament, the amount of time you have, or the need to deal with anger, pain, or some other specific health problem like insomnia. (See Chapter 2 for a listing of health problems that respond to meditation.)

These meditations can be used in a variety of circumstances: walking in a park, on a break at work, sitting in your backyard, listening to music, riding a train or bus, in doctors' waiting rooms, and in hundreds of other circumstances. Below is a short description of each meditation. These alternate meditation exercises supplement, but shouldn't entirely replace, your daily sitting meditation routine, which remains the foundation of your practice.

- **Walking meditation** is a healthy activity that combines two very powerful forms of stress reduction: physical exercise and meditation.

- **Zen breathing exercises** combine an awareness of breath with various insightful sayings or symbolic phrases. Meditation that is focused through the prism of these guidewords can help produce insight.

- **Yoga Complete Breath** is a method of yoga breathing that originated in ancient India and has benefited many people for thousands of years.

- **Well-Being** is a very simple meditation exercise. It is a welcome antidote to other more complicated techniques with long lists of instructions.

- **Pebble Meditation** is a meditation technique that promotes feelings of happiness and peace, and can easily be practiced by children as well as adults.

- **Meditation on the Whole Person** can enlarge your awareness of the present to include your entire body, feelings, perceptions of the surrounding environment, thoughts, and consciousness.

- **The Five Remembrances** is an exercise in understanding impermanence, motivating right action, and reducing the fear and sadness associated with illness, loss, and death.

- **Meditations for transforming anger and pain** can help you reduce these common forms of suffering.

- **Music meditation** and **music therapy** use music as a doorway to meditation and healing.

- **Mindful modes** are examples of special opportunities to practice mindfulness. This includes mindful modes of eating, exercising, spending time with a pet, driving, having sex, and working.

- **Meditations for a good night's sleep** reveals how to use meditation techniques to avoid insomnia.

- **The Stress Reliever physicians can teach in their office** is a stress-relieving meditation exercise that can easily be communicated to patients during a brief medical office visit. This is a good way for physicians and other healthcare providers to begin to teach meditation to their patients.

WALKING MEDITATION

Walking meditation involves focusing your entire attention on the movements of your body while walking. It is one of the best ways to link your mind to an awareness of what's going on in the rest of your body. Try not to think or talk while walking—just be hyperaware of the act of walking. Maintaining that focused awareness for any length of time requires concentration.

Try to practice walking meditation for fifteen to forty-five minutes several times a week.

1. **Choose an object to focus on.** The most common object of awareness during walking meditation is the feet. You might concentrate your entire awareness on just the soles of your feet. Feel the bottom of your feet gently grip the ground. Your feet may seem to "kiss" the ground with each step. Each step is a "quantum of nowness," a moment in time. Walk with spine aligned, head held high, and shoulders back. Be aware of your steps being very balanced and sure.

   Alternatively, you can focus awareness on other sensations while walking: like the feel of the movements of your legs, the feel of your fingers moving through the air, the swing of your arms, the smell of the air, or listening (without thinking) to the ambient background sounds. But, you can't concentrate on all of these things at once. So pick whatever focus works for you at the time.

2. **Enjoy each step.** Thich Nhat Hanh's book *The Long Road Turns to Joy: A Guide to Walking Meditation* (Parallax Press, 1996) is a wonderful reference for learning walking meditation. He writes,

   > We walk slowly, in a relaxed way, keeping a light smile on our lips. When we practice this way, we feel deeply at ease, and our steps are those of the most secure person on earth. All our sorrows and anxieties drop away, and peace and joy fill our hearts. Anyone can do it. It takes only a little time, a little mindfulness, and the wish to be happy. [Nhat Hanh adds] Why rush? Our final destination will only be the graveyard. Why not walk in the direction of life, enjoying peace in the moment with each step? There is no need to struggle. Enjoy each step. We have already arrived.

3. **Be mindful of your breath.** Be mindful of your breath while walking, but don't try to control it. You can harmonize your breath with your steps by noticing how many steps you take during your in-breath, and how many steps you take during your out-breath. I find this method particularly compelling when I am walking up flights of stairs. Counting steps like this helps me fully concentrate on each step, one at a time.

Another way to link your breath to the rhythm of your steps is by using the AH-OM mantra in the following way:

- On your in-breath, silently recite the sound of "AH" with each step.

- On your out-breath, hear "OM" with each step.

Hence, while inhaling you are silently saying "AH, AH, AH, AH" in time with the rhythm of your steps. During your out-breath hear the sound of "OM, OM, OM, OM" in time with your steps.

Alternatively, you can substitute other mantras. Instead of saying "AH-OM," you might recite the following mantra: *"Baba Nam Kevalam"* (pronounced like Bah-bah Nahm Kay-vuh-lum). This is a traditional mantra used in Ananda Marga meditation (an international spiritual practice and social service organization that was started in India in 1955). One translation of this Sanskrit mantra is "love is all there is." It is a musical-sounding mantra, almost like singing a song. I like to chant this mantra silently during walking meditation because it is very effective in helping to suppress the thinking mind.

- On your in-breath silently say, *"Ba-ba Nam."* Say this phrase in rhythm with your steps, at a pace of one step per syllable.

- On your out-breath say, *"Ke-va-lam"* in rhythm with your steps.

Putting a silent one-count rest between each phrase will give your steps a more even rhythm. Silently chant, *"Ba-ba-Nam"* (rest), *"Ke-va-lam"* (rest).

MORE VARIATIONS

During walking meditation you may want to recite spiritual poems (also called gathas) in time with your steps. This practice can help generate insight to transform negative states of mind. "The Five Insights" (page 195) and "Watering the Seeds" (page 196) are two of my favorite gathas to recite during walking meditation. The possible variations are endless, however. For example,

- You might just try silently chanting the word "now" with each step. This reminds you that each step is a moment of present awareness.

- *The Long Road Turns to Joy* contains several other examples of good walking meditation gathas. Another favorite of mine is Thich Nhat Hanh's poem "I Have Arrived":

I have arrived.
I am home
in the here, in the now.
I am solid. I am free.
In the ultimate I dwell.

Repeat this poem while walking slowly. Silently recite one three-word phrase with each step. If you prefer faster walking, say one word per step and place a silent "rest" count between each three-word phrase. Another variation is to recite the first line of the poem twice, and then recite the second line twice, and repeat just that much as you walk slowly.

The meaning of this poem is deep and subtle. "I have arrived. I am home" means that when we fully live in the moment, we can stop striving and relax, because we have already arrived in that place of peace, joy, and freedom. "I am solid" sounds contradictory to the Buddhist teaching that all things are "empty." But, being solid refers here to the stability that comes from being grounded in the solid wisdom that guides us along our life path. "In the ultimate I dwell" refers to dwelling happily in the wonders of the present. In that ultimate dimension we are free from fear because, though all things transform, nothing ever totally ceases to exist. (See pages 164 and 170 for more on the concepts of "emptiness" and the "ultimate dimension.")

THOUGHTS

Meditation is always about awareness of the present without thinking. During walking meditation thoughts will occur from time to time. As soon as you notice you are thinking, simply let the thoughts fade into the background (like the sound of the wind rustling through the leaves in the trees) while you gently redirect your awareness back to your mantra and your steps. Endeavoring to avoid naming things you see along the walking path will help you avoid lapsing into thought.

WHERE TO WALK

Almost any path can be a place to practice walking meditation. Either a quiet city park or a lonely dirt road work great. Walking around the block, or back and forth along a quiet neighborhood street can work just as well. It is best not to attempt walking meditation on a crowded city street; you need to think too much to stay safe from cars, and other people may try to talk to you, thereby interrupting the meditation. Elaborate circular walking paths called labyrinths have been constructed by people of all faiths for thousands of years; they can also be special places to practice walking meditation. For an example of one see Figure 2 below. A labyrinth near you can be located by going to the World-Wide Labyrinth Locator at the following website: wwll.veriditas.labyrinth society.org.

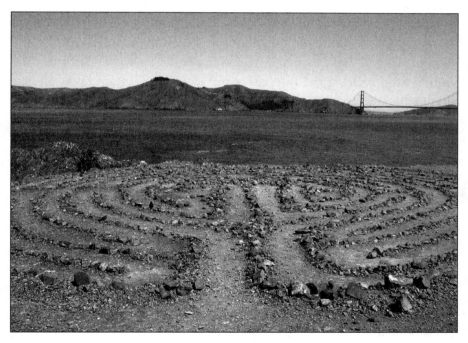

FIGURE 2. Land's End Labyrinth near San Francisco.

The Land's End Labyrinth pictured above is perched on a plateau off San Francisco's Coastal Trail and has a magnificent view of the Golden Gate Bridge.

Walking meditation is usually done outside, but may also be done indoors. For indoor walking meditation, try walking with very slow steps in a circular fashion around the perimeter of a large room. Take just one step with each in-breath, and one step with each out-breath. Later, if you feel like walking faster, take two steps with each in-breath, and two steps per out-breath.

WALKING THE PATH

I like walking meditation because it combines doing something healthy for your body with doing something healthy for your mind and spirit. If you notice any discomfort in your legs or back, simply regard it as "the taste of living," and be happy you are still able to experience it. Forming a slight smile with your lips (and eyes) while walking can secondarily increase your feeling of happiness.

It's okay to stop walking every now and then and just appreciate what is happening while standing still. You can pay attention to the scene in front of you, without thinking about it. Nonjudgmentally, you simply observe what is happening. If you want to listen to the surrounding sounds, stop reciting the internal mantra, while maintaining awareness of your breath.

Walking together arm in arm or holding hands with a friend is a great way to share the walking meditation experience with someone without talking. Walking meditation done with a group of people helps you feel your interconnectedness with other people, and how we are like separate water droplets in a great river of humanity. When I am in a large group of people doing walking meditation together, I often feel as if I am one little cell within a huge, multicellular organism (perhaps a giant caterpillar) moving slowly and mindfully down the path.

You can practice walking meditation while you walk your dog. But, you should stay conscious of what the dog is doing. So, while you are walking, keep your dog's movements within the field of your awareness without thinking about what the dog is doing. Or you might make awareness of the dog the main focus of your meditation for part of the walk.

When walking outside, it helps to often walk the same route, so you learn how long it takes to make a complete lap or loop along your route.

Then, if you have to be somewhere after walking meditation, you won't have the stress of keeping track of time while you are walking. Remember not to hurry along the path; you have already arrived.

Go outside and practice walking meditation right now!

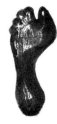

ZEN BREATHING EXERCISES

Using breath as a focus for meditation has advantages. After a few breaths you stop the discursive thinking that goes on inside your head and quickly link your mind to your body in the present. If you aren't always reciting the AH-OM mantra, you can then incorporate into your meditation other phrases and gathas that quiet your mind and help remind you of insights like impermanence, interconnectedness, nonattachment, and compassion.

THE SUTRA ON MINDFUL BREATHING

This breathing exercise, also called the Full Awareness of Breathing, is one of the most famous discourses taught by the Buddha. The sutra was memorized by his disciples and later translated from Sanskrit into Chinese by Gunabhadra in 443 C.E. Thich Nhat Hanh's translation from Chinese into English, on the following page, comes from lecture notes presented at the 2006 Breath of the Buddha Retreat at Plum Village.

In this sutra, Buddha describes a long series of breathing exercises, which first put your mind in touch with your breath, and then your whole body, while generating a feeling of relaxation, happiness, and peace. These exercises also help you gain insight into the root causes of negative feelings, and then transform them.

Memorizing all these breathing exercises is challenging. So they can be read by a leader while other meditators practice. The leader recites each pair of exercises one at a time. Then there is time for those assembled to practice each exercise in silent meditation for a couple of minutes before the group leader recites the next pair of breathing-exercise guidewords. This process is repeated until all sixteen pairs are completed. If practicing these exercises by yourself, you can read each pair of sentences and then practice the exercise for a minute or two before reading the next pair of sentences. (Italicized phrases within parentheses are clarifications that I have added.)

The Sutra

1. Skillfully, he practices breathing in, fully aware of his in-breath.
   Skillfully, he practices breathing out, fully aware of his out-breath.

2. Skillfully, he practices breathing in a long or a short breath, fully aware of his long or short breath.
   Skillfully, he practices breathing out a long or a short breath, fully aware of his long or short breath (*this means stay concentrated on the entire duration of the breath all the way through*).

3. Skillfully, he practices breathing in, fully aware of his whole body.
   Skillfully, he practices breathing out, fully aware of his whole body.

4. Skillfully, he practices breathing in, relaxing his whole body.
   Skillfully, he practices breathing out, relaxing his whole body.

5. Skillfully, he practices breathing in, experiencing joy.
   Skillfully, he practices breathing out, experiencing joy (*transform neutral feelings*).

6. Skillfully, he practices breathing in, experiencing happiness.
   Skillfully, he practices breathing out, experiencing happiness.

7. Skillfully, he practices breathing in, aware of his feelings.
   Skillfully, he practices breathing out, aware of his feelings (*particularly paying attention to any negative feelings that may be present*).

8. Skillfully, he practices breathing in, calming of his feelings.
   Skillfully, he practices breathing out, calming of his feelings (*smile to the feeling*).

9. Skillfully, he practices breathing in, aware of his mind.

    Skillfully, he practices breathing out, aware of his mind *(observe states of mind, meaning perceptions, thoughts, feelings, in order to see deeply and nonjudgmentally into the mind's activities)*.

10. Skillfully, he practices breathing in, gladdening his mind.

    Skillfully, he practices breathing out, gladdening his mind *(watering the good seeds)*.

11. Skillfully, he practices breathing in, concentrating his mind.

    Skillfully, he practices breathing out, concentrating his mind *(recalling the importance of concentration to the process of meditation)*.

12. Skillfully, he practices breathing in, liberating his mind.

    Skillfully, he practices breathing out, liberating his mind *(meditation generates a feeling of freedom)*.

13. Skillfully, he practices breathing in, contemplating impermanence.

    Skillfully, he practices breathing out, contemplating impermanence.

14. Skillfully, he practices breathing in, contemplating letting go.

    Skillfully, he practices breathing out, contemplating letting go *(let go of craving and clinging)*.

15. Skillfully, he practices breathing in, contemplating non-desire *(nonattachment)*.

    Skillfully, he practices breathing out, contemplating non-desire.

16. Skillfully, he practices breathing in, contemplating cessation *(of suffering)*.

    Skillfully, he practices breathing out, contemplating cessation *(of suffering)*.

From *The Sutra on Mindful Breathing* translated by Thich Nhat Hanh, 2006, used with permission of Parallax Press, Berkeley, CA; www.parallax.org.

BUDDHA'S BREATHING EXERCISES

It is difficult for lay practitioners to memorize an entire set of sixteen breathing exercises. So Buddha also taught a much shorter series of exercises called Buddha's Breathing Exercises that are easier to memorize, and if applied correctly, produce many of the same benefits.

As described by Thich Nhat Hanh in his book *Present Moment Wonderful Moment,* this breathing exercise is based on five pairs of guidewords: "in/out," "deep/slow," "calm/ease," "smile/release," and "present moment/wonderful moment." The first guideword (or words) of each pair is spoken silently, while you also concentrate on your in-breath. The second guideword of each pair is spoken silently while you focus on your out-breath. Phrases inside the parentheses below are my own clarifications about the meaning of the guidewords.

Say during your in-breath:	Say during your out-breath:
In *(I am aware of my in breath)*	Out *(I am aware of my out breath)*
Deep *(breath)*	Slow *(breathing)*
Calm *(stop hurrying and center yourself)*	Ease *(the muscles of the body)*
Smile	Release *(the negative feelings)*
Present moment	Wonderful moment

Follow the instructions below and try practicing a whole set of Buddha's Breathing Exercises right now.

1. **In/Out.** Sit comfortably on a chair or on a cushion. Close your eyes, and gently bring your attention to your breath. The first pair of guidewords is in/out, which help link your mind to your breath.

   • While breathing in, say the word "in."

   • And while breathing out, silently say the word "out."

   Or, you could say to yourself:

   • "Breathing in, I am aware of my in-breath."

   • "Breathing out, I am aware of my out-breath."

After a couple of minutes, move to the next pair of guidewords.

2. **Deep/Slow.** This reminds you to stay focused on your in-breath and out-breath all the way through, as your breath naturally becomes deeper and slower.

- On your in-breath, silently say the word "deep."
- On your out-breath, say the word "slow."

After a couple of minutes, go on to the third exercise.

3. **Calm/Ease.** "Calm" means to stop hurrying, peacefully center yourself, and align your body. "Ease" means to relax the muscles of the body. Perform a body scan.

- With each in-breath, say the word "calm" and feel your calm center and the "aliveness" within your body.
- With each out-breath, say the word "ease" while you relax each part of the body, from the top of your head down to the tips of your toes, one level at a time.

This will take several minutes. When you have finished an entire body scan using the guidewords "calm/ease," then go on to the next exercise.

4. **Smile/Release.** With each in-breath you are reminded to place a smile on your face, to gladden your mind and help you feel fresher. With each out-breath release any negative feelings.

- On your in-breath, silently say the word "smile."
- On your out-breath, say the word "release."

Remember to smile with your eyes as well as your lips. Become aware of any negative feelings you may have—whether it may be a feeling of anger, frustration, sorrow, fear, anxiety, or just boredom. Then, during your out-breath, release these negative feelings. You might also say to yourself something like this:

- "Breathing in, I smile to my negative feelings."
- "Breathing out, I release my negative feelings."

After you practice releasing your negative feelings for several minutes, go on to the last exercise.

5. **Present moment/Wonderful moment.** You might say to yourself something like this:

- "Breathing in, I am aware of the present moment. I am staying in the moment."

- "Breathing out, I enjoy this wonderful moment. I am dwelling in the wonders of the here and now."

I usually practice Buddha's Breathing Exercises as a sitting meditation exercise. But, these exercises can also be practiced while doing routine daily activities, like getting dressed in the morning, or while walking, doing housework, or yard work. While doing these routine activities, if I am already mindful of my breath, I often just start by practicing the third pair of guidewords: "calm/ease." This reminds me to stop hurrying, return to the calm island inside myself, and ease the muscles of my body. I may recite this pair of guidewords for a few minutes and then go on to the next pair: "smile/release." This puts a smile on my face, and for several minutes with each out-breath I release any negative feelings I may have. Then I go on to "present moment/wonderful moment." After enjoying the present moment for a couple of minutes, I may repeat all three pairs of breathing exercises all over again.

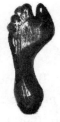

YOGA COMPLETE BREATH

Yoga Complete Breath is a breathing technique that expands your lungs to their fullest capacity. By doing this meditation breathing exercise, you can enhance your mindfulness of breath, center yourself, relax your mind, cleanse your lungs, and energize your body.

For people with chronic lung disease or asthma, this is a way of improving their respiratory capacity. Maynard Ferguson, the famous high-note jazz trumpet player, was known for using yoga breathing exercises to help build his phenomenal trumpet range.

While sitting upright with aligned posture, practice breathing as noted below.

1. **During the in-breath:** Try to do the following three steps as one smooth, continuous breath, without any separation between the steps.

   • Expand your diaphragm by pushing the abdomen forward as you breathe in.

   • Expand the ribs sideways while still breathing in. (You will notice your abdomen will automatically go inward slightly.)

   • Lift up your upper chest and shoulders while inhaling the last portion of your in-breath.

2. **During the out-breath:** Do the following three steps as one smooth, continuous breath, without any separation between the steps.

   • Lower your shoulders and shoulder blades slightly.

   • Let the chest and ribs relax as the air automatically goes out.

   • When all the air seems to be out, push in the abdomen slightly to expel any air remaining in the lungs.

While doing this exercise, maintain an upright and aligned posture with an open throat, so as to not impede the free flow of air into the lungs. Repeat this exercise as many times as you like. It only takes three breaths to make a positive difference to the way you feel.

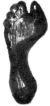

WELL-BEING

Well-Being is a very simple sitting-meditation breathing exercise I created. Here "well" stands for all the positive mental states, and "being" means to be here now.

• On your in-breath, silently say to yourself the word "well."

• On your out-breath, say the word "being."

Silently chant this simple mantra, while you are aware of breathing in and breathing out, for fifteen to twenty minutes. When you notice any thoughts occurring, gently direct your attention back to the mantra "well-being." This exercise generates a peaceful and pleasant state of mind that remains focused on the present.

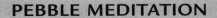

PEBBLE MEDITATION

Pebble Meditation was developed by Thich Nhat Hanh as a meditation that can easily be done by children. But, adults can also benefit from it just as much as kids.

Start this meditation by taking four pebbles and placing them next to you on your left side. Then, pick up the pebbles one at a time, while being mindful of the following images or guidewords: "flower," "mountain," "still water," and "space." As you hold one pebble in your hand, breathe three breaths while meditating on each guideword and imagining an associated image. When you have completed the meditation with one pebble, put it down on your right, and then pick up the next pebble, as you breathe three more times with the next guideword and image in mind.

Find a quiet place to sit, and begin.

1. **First Pebble: Flower.** This image represents freshness. While holding the first pebble in your hand, you say to yourself,

   • "Breathing in, I see myself as a flower. Breathing out, I feel fresh."

   Do this three times, put the pebble down, and pick up the next pebble.

2. **Second Pebble: Mountain.** This image represents solidity, stability, dependability. While holding the second pebble in your hand, you say to yourself,

   • "Breathing in, I see myself as a mountain. Breathing out, I feel solid."

   Do this three times, put the pebble down, and pick up the next pebble.

3. **Third Pebble: Still Water.** This image represents peace, calmness, and serenity. When you are peaceful and calm, you can reflect things as they are (without distortion); as if you are a still, reflecting pool of water. While holding the third pebble in your hand, you say to yourself,

- "Breathing in, I see myself as still water. Breathing out, I feel peaceful."

Do this three times, put the pebble down, and pick up the last pebble.

4. **Fourth Pebble: Space.** This image represents space and freedom—space from having too many projects, possessions, or angry emotions crowding out your freedom. While holding the fourth pebble in your hand, you say to yourself,

- "Breathing in, I see myself as space. Breathing out, I feel free."

Place the last pebble down to your right.

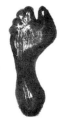

MEDITATION ON THE WHOLE PERSON

When practicing the AH-OM Breath meditation, one focuses awareness on the breath and the sound of the mantra. The Meditation on the Whole Person exercise allows you to expand your field of awareness to include your entire self and beyond. Buddhism divides the entity that is "the person" into five components or "aggregates": the body (also called form); feelings (joy, sorrow, neutrality, energetic, tiredness, anticipation, anxiety, fear, disgust, shame, sympathy, freshness, and so on); perceptions (sounds, temperature, smells, tastes, sights); mental formations (thoughts); and consciousness (awareness). Each of the five aggregates is continually changing—some changing quickly, others more slowly.

To help understand the constantly changing nature of the person, or so-called self, Buddha taught: meditate by focusing your awareness on each of the five aggregates, one at a time.

1. **Aggregate one: Meditate on the body.** While sitting, begin this meditation with the usual AH-OM Breath meditation technique described in Chapter 1. Then allow the sound of the mantra to fade into the background, focusing your awareness completely on breathing in and breathing out—the so-called breath-body. After you are fully concentrated on your breath, expand the field of your awareness to include the rest of your body by doing a whole-body scan. You might start at

the top and work your way down, one body part at a time. With each in-breath, focus your awareness on one part of the body and feel the "aliveness," or "life energy," within that body part. With each out-breath, try to relax or ease the body part. Spend a minute or two practicing each step listed below.

- Beginning on your in-breath, concentrate on the feeling of "aliveness" in your scalp and forehead. With each out-breath, feel your forehead and scalp muscles relax and flatten.

- Then, in the same manner, scan your face, jaw, and tongue. Feel the "aliveness" there during your in-breath. And feel the relaxation there during your out-breath. Do this for several breaths, while your eyelid muscles relax and become flatter, and your jaw and tongue become looser.

- Now pay close attention to the sensations in your neck and shoulders. Feel your neck muscles become looser and your shoulders start to drop lower as your muscles become less bunched. After a few breaths, move on to the next region of the body.

- During your in-breath, feel the "life energy" in your arms, hands, and fingers. With each out-breath feel your hands become less clenched as your fingers float free. After a minute or so, shift attention to the core of your body.

- Focus on the alignment of your spine and the sensations in your upper and lower back. You may want to stretch and twist your back a bit in order to better align and loosen any stiffness in it, and unlock (or pop) any stuck facet joints in the spine.

- Next, scan your entire chest, abdomen, and pelvis. Enjoy the outward and inward movements of your chest. Feel your diaphragm expand as your breath becomes progressively deeper and slower. On your in-breath, feel the sensations inside your belly. With each out-breath feel the sphincter muscles of the pelvis become more relaxed.

- Lastly, focus your attention on your legs, feet, and toes. If you notice any pain or tightness in your thighs or calves, try to progressively relax that area with each out-breath. Feel as if the breath is going in and out of your feet. Wiggle your toes a little as if they were your little wings. Then, after you have completed a full body scan, begin to meditate on your feelings. Now move on to aggregate two.

2. **Aggregate two: Meditate on your feelings.** As you breathe in and out, notice whatever feeling or emotion you are experiencing right now.

  • If you are having a positive feeling, just "groove on it." If you are in a neutral state, you might try to "gladden" your mind by drawing the corners of your lips into a slight Buddha-like smile. Begin to feel fresher, lighter, and happier as you breathe in and out for a couple of minutes.

  • If you are in a negative emotional state, such as feeling anger, fear, nervousness, or sadness, you might calm and "embrace" it by saying, "Breathing in, I am aware anger (fear or sadness) is inside me. Breathing out, I smile to my anger (fear or sadness)." When you feel the negative feelings "lighten up" after a few minutes (or more), it's time to move to the next exercise.

3. **Aggregate three: Meditate on your perceptions.** We become aware of our perceptions through our five senses.

  • First, become aware of the external sounds you hear, but don't think about, label, identify, or name the sounds you are hearing, as this would trigger a thinking process. Just notice the quality of the different sounds as they "play with your ears."

  • Next, notice what aromas can be perceived by your nose, and then what tastes can be sensed by your tongue. Sometime try this exercise while mindfully eating food or drinking juice, tea, or coffee. You can then notice so much more perceptual input arising from your sense of taste and smell. Meditate by focusing on what you can smell during your in-breath, and taste during your out-breath. Feel the textures as you chew and swallow.

  • Next, become aware of what sensations your skin and fingers are feeling: temperature, humidity, breezes, pain, contours, and textures.

- Last, notice what perceptions are entering your mind through the eyes. At first, don't open your eyes. Just notice the multicolored, changing patterns that can be perceived behind your closed eyelids. After a minute, open your eyes halfway and then all the way and look around you. Notice what sights and colors can be perceived, without thinking about what you see. Avoid labeling or naming what you see, because that often initiates thinking. Just be non-judgmentally aware of what is there. After absorbing those sights for a little while, move on to aggregate four.

4. **Aggregate four: Meditate on mental formations.** Here, be aware of your thoughts without becoming attached to them.

   - Feel the thoughts forming and changing. Notice how one thought or perception triggers the next thought. Don't react to the thoughts with like or dislike, judgment, or reflection. It is as if you are on a bridge watching the river of your thoughts flow by. After a couple of minutes, move on to aggregate five.

5. **Aggregate five: Meditate on consciousness.** Consciousness is awareness of yourself and your surroundings in a remembered present. This phenomenon that we call consciousness requires millions of connections between nerve cells in various parts of the brain to form reverberating circuits. Meditation can bring these reverberating circuits into a more coherent harmony. Now to meditate on consciousness . . .

   - First, focus your concentration on being alive in this place, in this moment. Become very still and just be aware that you are aware.

   - Try to keep focused on what it feels like to maintain that state of pure awareness of the present, without thinking. Stay concentrated like this for a few minutes.

Like a river that looks fairly similar from day to day, the components of a person seem to have a kind of continuity over time. But, like the water in the river, the pieces of your whole person are actually constantly changing. By doing this meditation, you can notice the five constantly changing rivers of your whole person.

You will also notice there is only so much you can be aware of at any one time. So, while you can greatly expand your awareness of what is happening in the present, your view of your present reality is always somewhat limited. However, Meditation on the Whole Person allows the field of your awareness to expand to include much more of what is happening in the present. Eventually, it all becomes "one big happening."

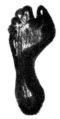

THE FIVE REMEMBRANCES

The Buddha told his monks to practice meditating every day on what he called The Five Remembrances. He asked them to contemplate these harsh realities in an unsentimental, unflinching fashion. The first four remembrances remind us of some inescapable causes of suffering in everyone's life, like illness and death. Buddha asked his students to recall and recite these truths on a regular basis for this reason: when you become convinced that these eventual outcomes are inescapable, it is liberating because you stop constantly worrying about how to prevent these natural outcomes. In addition, this exercise can contribute to your happiness because, if you still have your life, basic health, and any living friends and family, reciting the Five Remembrances prevents you from taking these wondrous things for granted.

The fifth remembrance reminds you of the reason for practicing the way of wisdom, morality, and meditation (the three keys to enlightenment discussed in Chapter 3). It is because—despite existing in a constantly changing world—this practice gives you a "grounded" sense of stability and peace.

The Five Remembrances can either be done as a solo silent sitting meditation or as a group meditation. If done as a group, a leader will recite each remembrance once and then the group silently contemplates the truth of these words as they calm their emotions by peacefully paying attention to their in-breath and out-breath. If you practice this meditation alone, say each remembrance silently to yourself. Then mindfully breathe in and out three slow breaths before turning your attention to the next remembrance.

The Five Remembrances

1. I am of the nature to grow old.
   There is no way to escape growing old.

2. I am of the nature to have ill health.
   There is no way to escape having ill health.

3. I am of the nature to die.
   There is no way to escape death.

4. All that is dear to me and everyone I love are of the nature to change.
   There is no way to escape being separated from them.

5. I inherit the results of my actions in body, speech, and mind.
   My actions are the ground on which I stand.

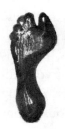

MEDITATIONS FOR TRANSFORMING ANGER

Anger is one of the most common causes of human suffering. It is amazing how quickly anger can arise to disrupt your peace and happiness. As an analogy, consider a fluffy cloud serenely floating in the sky. It looks so calm and tranquil; but, under certain conditions, that same cloud can rapidly issue forth an outrageously loud crack of thunder and a fierce, energy-charged lightning bolt that can strike a person dead in an instant. Similarly, a human can feel peaceful one minute, but then something might occur the next minute that can throw them into a rage. For instance, I have had the experience of feeling good, when suddenly something occurs at work, or perhaps my daughter or wife says something, that rapidly throws me into a state of anger and makes me feel just terrible.

The section "Feelings" in Chapter 7 explains why anger can manifest in us so quickly. How this reaction can, in a split second, be so swiftly triggered by the neurological pathways that go directly from the eye or the ear through a little group of neurons in the center of the brain called the amygdala, which then reflexively triggers a whole set of emotional responses without requiring any involvement of higher cortical regions in the brain.

No matter how enlightened we are, the seed of anger remains within all of us. It waits there ready to manifest in our consciousness when certain conditions arise. When the seed of anger is activated, it often manifests in a way that we want to punish the other person for daring to cause us to suffer. Then you retaliate and escalate up the ladder of suffering, and you both suffer more. Fortunately, there are skillful means that can transform anger and protect us from the devastating damage that anger causes in us and in other people to whom we might direct an angry reaction.

PUT THE ANGER IN A DIFFERENT PERSPECTIVE

In his book *Buddhist Meditation and Depth Psychology* (Pariyatti Press, 1994), psychiatrist Douglas Burns describes that when a person is angry their first inclination is to direct an angry response to the other person, usually making the situation worse. But, if we take a moment to reflect on our anger, we can interrupt the amplification of anger's negative effects. Dr. Burns writes,

> The Buddhist approach is to turn attention to the real problem— the anger. One reflects, *I am angry . . . It is real; it is intense . . . It is a feeling . . . It has no reality outside my own consciousness . . . Like all feelings it will soon diminish . . . I experience it but am not compelled to act on it.* With practice one finds that though anger still arises, its effect is diminished.

When you find yourself getting mad at someone, it is helpful to put the situation in a larger perspective by reciting this Thich Nhat Hanh poem entitled "Seeing Emotions Through the Eyes of Impermanence":

Angry in the ultimate dimension*
I close my eyes and look deeply.
Three hundred years from now
where will you be and where shall I be?

---

* See page 170 for an explanation of the ultimate dimension.

It is hard to stay mad at someone when you think about the meaning of this poem.

COOL THE FLAMES

Anger can be calmed and transformed into something more positive and healing by using meditation techniques described by Thich Nhat Hanh in his book *Anger: Wisdom for Cooling the Flames* (Riverhead Books, 2001).

Thich Nhat Hanh teaches that when you notice anger is inside of you, treat your anger like a mother treats her baby. When a baby is suffering, the mother stops everything else she is doing and immediately starts to cradle and rock the baby in her arms. And even before the mother understands why the baby is crying, the baby senses the love and concern from the mother's soothing touch, and the baby suffers less and may stop crying.

Treat your anger as if it were your baby. Don't ignore it. It is your reaction to something that triggered the "seed of anger," which is in all of us. Immediately stop everything else you are doing, and start to lovingly cradle your anger with mindfulness. Don't direct the heat of your anger outward, because punishing the other person is self-punishment. Treat yourself with compassion, and try the following:

1. **Calm your anger.** The first step is to cool the flames of your anger by practicing sitting meditation or walking meditation for at least fifteen minutes.

2. **If needed, calm your anger further.** You might further calm the anger by repeating this simple meditation breathing exercise for several minutes:
   - "Breathing in, I know anger is in me. Breathing out, I smile to take care of my anger."

3. **Gain insight into the source of your anger.** Then, after your emotions have calmed down, and your mind is very still, continue to practice sitting or walking meditation for another thirty minutes or more. This often produces insights that allow you to understand the roots of your anger.

THE THREE SENTENCES

If the process described above sufficiently resolves and completely calms your anger, you can leave it at that. But let's say you have been practicing sitting and walking meditation, and by the next day you are still angry. Then, Thich Nhat Hanh recommends that you take the process one step further by talking to the person whose actions triggered your anger. He says, after you have cooled the flames of anger in yourself, you have a duty to let the other person know that you are still angry by talking (or writing) to them the very next day if possible. Let the other person know you are suffering, but you must do this using calm, loving speech.

You might say something like this: "What you did hurt me a lot. I would like to make a plan to meet with you in a couple of days when we both have the time to talk and can discuss it calmly and peacefully." The other person may ask you to talk about it right now. But don't do that because you are not calm enough. Your anger will be expressed in harsh speech, creating defensiveness in the other person, which will only make coming to a resolution much harder. Wait until you have had time to calm down and meditate about the situation. Consider the possibility that you may have misperceived the other person's intentions.

Thich Nhat Hanh suggests that when the two of you finally get together for the deeper discussion, the following three basic sentences should be communicated to the other person. (You might write down these three sentences on a card, and keep the card in your wallet as a handy reference for when anger arises.)

1. **Sentence One:** "Darling, I am angry, I am suffering, and I want you to know it." Use of the word "Darling" or some other term of endearment is optional. The main thing is to acknowledge to yourself that you are suffering and let the other person know it too. Be as specific as you can in telling the other person exactly what their action was that precipitated your anger. You might add, "I don't know why you have done such a thing to me." Remember to use loving speech. Don't characterize them as a "bad person."

2. **Sentence Two:** "I am trying my best to handle my anger." This second sentence means that I am endeavoring to refrain from acting out of anger. I am practicing sitting and walking meditation to embrace and cool my anger. I am trying not to blame anyone. I am looking deeply to see if there might be some misperception that triggered the anger, as there often is. This is also an indirect invitation to the other person to do the same, and to ask themselves what it was they may have done wrong.

   In order to look deeply, it helps to be mindful of the four insights of impermanence, interconnectedness, nonattachment, and compassion that were discussed in Chapter 3. Endeavor to apply the wisdom of these insights to this specific situation and to your feeling about the other person. Keep these insights constantly alive when you are meditating to transform your anger. Meditation, in this context, means to take the time to sit quietly and look deeply in order to accurately reflect on your relations with other people. When you truly understand how impermanent it all is—how eventually we lose all our possessions and all our loved ones—you will then have more compassion for the other person and for yourself. You will also be able to forgive the faults in the other person and in yourself. It is then easier to let go of past grudges, of feeling insulted or ignored, and of feelings like jealousy, greed, hatred, and fear.

3. **Sentence Three:** "Please help me understand." Here you are asking the other person to please explain why they said what they said, or did what they did (or didn't do), that caused your anger. You are asking the other person to help you to understand their point of view about why this happened. Often the other person's actions or apparent insensitivity has occurred as a result of their own fears and suffering. Have compassion for what they are experiencing.

   This third sentence is always the hardest one for us to say, because when we are angry at someone the usual tendency is to want to push that person away saying, "I don't need you." We are prideful, and when someone close to us says something that dares to make us suffer, we often react by turning our backs on them and blocking them out of our lives to prove we don't need them.

On the contrary, however, it is very important for us to look at them, and hear what their perceptions and intentions were. And you must communicate the same to them. "Please help me understand" means that you are asking the other person to help you suffer less by talking about whatever it was that triggered your anger. Therefore, you are not "papering over" or ignoring your differences but are instead trying to come to a mutual understanding or insight.

If you *can't* bring yourself to speak to the other person directly and calmly, then write down these statements on a piece of paper and deliver the written statement to them, or e-mail it to them. Even if the other person can't, or won't, respond to you, writing it down will help you to suffer less.

OTHER POSITIVE WAYS TO COMMUNICATE ANGER

When communicating to someone about the cause of your anger, don't use phrases that negatively characterize the other person, such as "Don't be such a jerk!" or "Why are you so insensitive?" This type of language will always make the situation worse. Talk with the other person using loving speech and deep listening. Author Marshall Rosenthal calls this type of speech "nonviolent communication." His book, *Nonviolent Communication: A Language of Life,* contains many suggestions about how to talk this way. If you speak in reproachful and blaming terms, it will wreck the chance for the clarity you are seeking. Even when there has developed a long-standing argument or grudge between people, the anger-management techniques described above can be used to skillfully start a process of forgiveness and "beginning anew."

Don't forget that the other person is suffering too. So, practice deep listening when the other person speaks. When they speak to you, don't interrupt their statement so it becomes like an argument. The other person's voice may be bitter, or sour, or full of blame. But just listen. You might say to them phrases such as "Please continue to speak" or "Please help me to understand." Encourage them to reveal details and unburden their whole heart. It is not easy, but we must listen very closely to things that are said and not said. Just by sympathetic listening you can help them reduce a lot of their suffering. If you recognize that you have been wrong, you can apologize right away. But if you still disagree with them, don't try to correct their misperceptions right away. Let some time pass. You can gently release some information to them about why they were wrong a little at a time, over the next few days.

When discussing your differences with someone don't be too attached to your own views. After both of you have heard each other, it is best not to debate your differences endlessly. Instead, let what you have heard mellow in the cauldron of meditation, so greater insight can later be realized and communicated. This process may need to continue over a long period of time, while two-way communication and negotiation takes place and your anger is repeatedly dissipated. It takes time for the flames of passion to cool. So don't expect instant transformation, even when a clear misperception has been corrected. It may take days before the feeling of the emotional reaction of anger totally subsides.

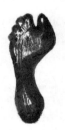

MEDITATIONS FOR TRANSFORMING PAIN

It is important to have an integrated approach to pain that employs any necessary medical workup to exclude serious conditions. If appropriate, employ therapies such as medication treatment, physical therapy, yoga, stretching, massage, chiropractic, or acupuncture as adjunctive ways to diminish pain. But, while these therapies are pretty good at relieving acute pain, they are often inadequate at treating chronic pain. People with chronic conditions like osteoarthritis of the knees and back, recurring headaches, a prior outbreak of shingles, or diabetic neuropathy have pain that modern medicine usually can't cure. However, meditation techniques can significantly reduce their pain and restore their quality of life.

SEPARATE THE PAIN FROM THE FEAR OF WHAT IT MEANS

The fear of what the pain means is often the most distressing thing about the pain. For example, we might fear that a mildly painful arthritic condition in the knees or hips could progress to a point where we wouldn't be able to walk well enough to get around or to do our job. Or we might fear that a minor chest pain or arm numbness could be due to an impending heart attack or stroke. In his book *Full Catastrophe Living*, Jon Kabat-Zinn writes, "Aversion to pain is really a misplaced aversion to suffering. Even a small pain can produce great suffering if we fear it means we have a tumor or some other frightening condition. That same pain can be seen as nothing at all, a minor ache or inconvenience, once we are reassured all the tests are negative and there is no chance that it is a sign of something serious."

Right now, in the present moment, if we can separate the sensation of pain itself from the fear of what it means, the pain is usually much more tolerable. So, let's start with the following steps:

1. **Practice a calming meditation technique.** Use AH-OM Breath meditation or Buddha's Breathing Exercises for fifteen to thirty minutes to reduce the fear, anxiety, and associated stress. After fear and anxiety are calmed, we are then better able to take the next step, which is to focus our attention directly on the pain.

2. **Breathe with the pain.** With this next breathing exercise, you're trying to get to know your pain better, rather than expecting to completely get rid of it. Research done at the University of Massachusetts Stress Reduction Clinic has found that meditation techniques can often reduce pain by 50 percent (which is pretty impressive as treatment for chronic, intractable pain).

   The following is an outline of a breathing exercise used at the clinic to help relieve pain. This technique is described in more detail in *Full Catastrophe Living*. When practicing this exercise, do so gently, without setting up a struggle between you and your pain, which would only create more tension and thereby more pain.

   • On your in-breath, imagine you are breathing in through the painful area of the body, as you focus your full awareness calmly and deeply on the painful sensation.

   • On your out-breath, imagine you are breathing out through a hole in the same part of the body. Each time you breathe out, release some of the tension and the pain.

- In turn, first feel your pain on the in-breath, then let go of tension as you smile to your pain on the out-breath. Feel the pain change as the rest of the body relaxes more with each out-breath.

The following is an alternate breathing exercise you can use to reduce pain. Focus on your breath and your pain as you silently say to yourself,

- "Breathing in, I am aware of my pain."
- "Breathing out, I smile to my pain."

As with the previous exercise, embrace the pain on your in-breath, and progressively relax the tension and ease the pain on your out-breath.

Try to "witness" the pain in a calm, nonjudgmental way. Don't say, "I hurt." You are not the pain. Instead, observe that the pain is something inside of you. Observe how it changes over time. Kabat-Zinn recommends asking ourselves, "How bad is it right now, in this very moment . . . In this moment is it tolerable? Is it okay?" He then provides the answer and a solution: "The chances are you will find that it is. The difficulty is that the next moment is coming, and the next, and you 'know' they are all going to be filled with more pain. The solution? Try taking each moment as it comes. Try to be 100 percent in the present in one moment, then do the same for the next, right through a forty-five-minute practice period, or until the intensity of the pain subsides."

3. **Focus on the pain-free body part using modeling meditation.** In order to reduce pain in one part of the body, I have found it also helps to try focusing your attention on how wonderful it is that the opposite part of your body (like the other knee or the rest of your back) is working well without pain. As a pain-reduction exercise, try modeling the movements of the painful body part after the movements of the opposite, normal body part. Practice modeling meditation for at least fifteen minutes a day. It's surprising how quickly this exercise can reduce the pain.

As a case in point, I used this technique to help me cope with a very painful common foot condition I had for months called plantar fasciitis. After trying several other treatments and shoe inserts, I wasn't making much progress. Then, as a thought experiment, I tried focusing my attention, not on the painful foot, but on observing how marvelously well my good foot moved when walking. I then simply asked my painful foot to walk more like my good foot. And the painful foot was almost immediately able to start walking with less of a limp and much less pain. I then repeated this modeling meditation exercise for about fifteen minutes every day until my foot eventually healed and the exercise was no longer necessary.

I think the reason this approach to pain reduction works has a lot to do with the capacity of the brain to rewire itself in response to repeated modeling stimuli. Neuroscientists call the capacity of the brain to change in this way "neuroplasticity," which is explained in more detail in Chapter 7, in the sections on "Consciousness" and "Learning and Wisdom."

4. **Your reaction to the pain is not the pain itself.** When mindfully working with your pain, be aware that all the thoughts and feelings you have about the pain are not the pain itself. They are reactions in your mind, which is unwilling to accept the pain and wants to be rid of it. When you come to see and feel what you are experiencing as pure sensation, you may see the thoughts about the sensations are actually making things worse. It is for this reason that Kabat-Zinn advises letting go of those thoughts, and try just accepting the painful condition for now, even if you hate the pain. He asks, "What about purposely stepping back from the hatred and anger and not judging things at all, just accepting them?" To paraphrase, you invite the thoughts and feelings about the pain into the field of your awareness and then intentionally let go of them, as you tune in to a sense of being complete in the present moment.

Remember to have compassion for yourself and your pain. Don't try too hard, and don't expect quick results. Regular practice, patience, and sustained concentration are necessary to make progress.

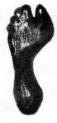

MUSIC MEDITATION

Music has deep effects on the mind. Listened to in a mindful way, music becomes a form of meditation. Music can also be used as music therapy to reduce stress, pain, and help heal the body of illness. In the foreword to Don Campbell's *Music: Physician for Times to Come* (Quest Books, 2000), Grammy Award–winning composer and musician Paul Winter wrote that through music "we can be brought back to 'beginner's mind,' with the child in each of us reawakened by our allurement to sound and our natural yearning to resonate with the world."

When listening to or making music, we are not just trying to get to the end of the piece. Instead, we are focused on the here-and-now, note-by-note experience. So, just like meditation, music can create a present-oriented state of mindfulness. Extraordinary saxophonist and jazz icon John Coltrane practiced meditation for many years, and you can hear a meditative quality in many of his musical improvisations.

Listening to music mindfully requires one to be totally concentrated on the sound of the music and the feel of the rhythm. Enjoy the melody, harmony, and any lyrics. Let the music take you on a journey. Pat your foot, clap your hands, snap your fingers, bob or tilt your head in time with the beat, or just "groove" with your whole body. Late jazz legend Duke Ellington used to invite his audiences to become more physically involved in his music by playfully telling them, "By routining one's finger-snapping and choreographing one's earlobe-tilting, one discovers that one can become as cool as one wishes to be."

Attending a live music concert can be an exciting, "moving" experience—like the time I went to see Denny Zeitlin's piano trio at the Jazz Bakery in Los Angeles. Partway through the concert, I looked around at the other audience members seated behind me. Everyone was wide-awake, but they all seemed like they were in a trance with eyes closed, lips in a half smile, and heads bobbing in time to the music. They were all "digging" the moment, using music as a focus for their meditation. They were "grooving in the eternal present," beat by beat, note by note, toe tap by toe tap.

EXERCISE IN MUSIC MEDITATION

Try this exercise in music meditation. Follow the instructions below while listening to a recording of some of your favorite relaxing music. It might be something like Mozart's *Piano Concerto No. 21 in C Major.* Or you could try this exercise while listening to the jazz ballad "Fantasy-land," included on Track 6 of the *Teaching Meditation* audio CD that accompanies this book. However, any music that you find beautiful and relaxing is fine.

1. Start to play the selected music.

2. Sit in a comfortable chair and close your eyes.

3. Center yourself and relax your breath.

4. Relax your forehead, jaw, and shoulder muscles.

5. Feel the cares of the world melt away, as your breath slows and your mind rests in the beauty of the present moment.

6. Keep your attention concentrated on the music, and let the sound of the music become the focus for your meditation.

7. Let the melody and harmony penetrate deeply into your "mind's ear."

8. Continue to pay attention to your breath while you breathe with the music. (This links your mind to your body and the music.)

9. Move your body in time to the rhythm of the music.

Instead of soft, relaxing music, you may choose to play a happy, upbeat piece of music. When your whole body is rocking and grooving, it produces a feeling of increased energy and joy.

Spend some time deeply listening to great music often. You will come to feel how music can be a doorway to greater happiness. It may even improve your physical health and spiritual well-being.

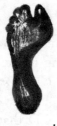

MUSIC THERAPY

In Greek mythology, Apollo was the sun god and the god of music. Apollo's mythological son, Asclepius, was the god of medicine. Asclepius often used music, diet, exercise, and spirituality as means of healing. Asclepius's son, Hippocrates, became the most celebrated physician in the ancient world. Historically, the ancient Greeks often used music as a healing art.

Music therapy is now a recognized academic field of research, with several universities offering advanced degrees in music therapy. Music therapists have a professional association, the American Music Therapy Association, which publishes and supports clinical research. Their website (www.musictherapy.org) has links to the *Journal of Music Therapy.*

Like other forms of meditation, music can elicit the relaxation response. Music therapy research has found that listening to certain types of music can lower blood pressure and heart rate, and reduce stress, anxiety, and pain, including postoperative pain and cancer pain.

Music can help improve mood, attentiveness, and activity level in patients who are cognitively impaired from previous strokes or Alzheimer's disease. I have seen this work in local nursing homes where a weekly concert from a local Dixieland band or a guitarist playing old familiar songs can bring back to life some of these otherwise withdrawn people, and have them smiling, singing, and tapping their feet.

Researchers at the University of California at Irvine found that ten minutes of listening to a Mozart piano concerto significantly improved the spatial IQ of test participants compared to controls. These researchers postulated that the complex patterns in Mozart's music helps organize the firing patterns of neurons in the cerebral cortex, especially strengthening creative right-brain processes associated with spatial-temporal reasoning.

While researching therapeutic effects of music, the late French physician and educator Alfred Tomatis often used music composed by Wolfgang Amadeus Mozart, an approach that he called the "Mozart effect." Music therapist Don Campbell, who wrote a book named *The Mozart Effect* (HarperCollins, 2001), claims Mozart's music is medicine for the body, mind, and soul. Campbell has also compiled a series of CDs entitled *Music for the Mozart Effect* (Spring Hill, 1998), which contains selections of music that work well as music therapy.

Musical styles other than classical Mozart can also produce beneficial effects. Which particular music selections work best as music therapy varies from person to person. It usually works best to find a musical style that the person already likes. Well-chosen familiar songs are usually the most evocative.

JAZZ

Dee Coulter is a neuroscience educator who specializes in the relationship between musical patterning and neurological development. She is quoted in *The Mozart Effect* as recommending jazz music "for optimal creativity, and for grappling with situations that do not lend themselves to simple linear solutions . . . It involves paying attention, while in a community, and being able to respond without being sure what's coming next."

Jazz proves that spontaneous recovery from unexpected events can be exciting and beautiful. Jazz has arguably been called America's only truly indigenous art form. It does make sense that jazz would have been invented in the United States, because a jazz band is a great metaphor for the ideals of the American democratic society. In a jazz band, everyone is given a chance to spontaneously and creatively "tell their own story." But they also have a shared responsibility to play their assigned role and be supportive of the other players in the group for the good of the overall sound.

In the December 2006 online edition of *JazzTimes* (www.JazzTimes.com), well-known jazz writer Nat Hentoff writes about the legacy of Louis Armstrong and his interest in music therapy. In Satchmo's name, the Louis and Lucille Armstrong Music Therapy Program was established in 1994 at the Beth Israel Medical Center in New York. Hentoff reports,

Throughout Beth Israel, staff members use music therapy on themselves . . . [to] manage their own stress and avoid burnout. The center offers music meditation for oncology nurses—group sessions where nurses sing and listen to live music . . . And every other week groups of medical residents convene in the center's music studios to play the drums, progressing from simple to more complex beats and working out their tension along the way.

CHANTING

Group chanting can have melody like other musical forms, or it can have no melody. But, all group chanting has a rhythmic feel that connects people closer together. Chanting has long been used as therapy for the soul in many religions. Examples include the tradition of the Gregorian chants in the Roman Catholic Church dating from the ninth and tenth centuries, and there is an even longer history of Jewish prayer chants. Chanting has also been used from ancient times in the Hindu and Buddhist traditions. While sitting in a meditation hall, I have been very moved by the powerful sound of hundreds of monks and nuns in ceremonial golden saffron robes chanting in unison the following well-known Sanskrit chant, done exactly the same way it has been done for more than 2,500 years:

> Gate gate paragate parasamgate bodhi svaha.
> Gate gate paragate parasamgate bodhi svaha.
> Gate gate paragate parasamgate bodhi svaha.

The mantra is rhythmically chanted in unison by the group, over and over, for several minutes. It roughly translates as follows: "Gone, gone, gone beyond, gone completely beyond, hail awakening." This mantra is contained in the Heart Sutra (one of the famous sermons given by the Buddha). Going "beyond" refers, in part, to going beyond seeing yourself and all things as separate, and awakening to the insight of interconnectedness.

BLUES

The blues is a vocal and instrumental form of music that strongly relates to people coping with physical and mental adversity. The late Jimmy

Cheatham, who co-led the Sweet Baby Blues Band, used to always say that blues, when played from the heart, could heal illness. There is something about hearing a person tell their story of hardship that is healing for the listener, the singer, and the other players in the band.

There is often a humorous or ironic element in blues' lyrics that also helps people cope with life's suffering. A good example is a song Jeannie and Jimmy Cheatham wrote called "Too Many Goodbyes." Recorded on their *Blues and the Boogie Masters* album, Jeannie, in a plaintive voice, sings,

> The doctor looks you in the eye.
> Says 'No more pork chops. Lord, no more pie.'
> Well, there's been too many good-byes in my life.

BE THE MUSIC

Listening to music is healing. But, imagine what might happen if you were actually making the music yourself and telling your own story. Another type of music therapy would then be occurring. It would be a here-and-now cooperative effort of your mind, body, and spirit to create your own personal work of art.

In fact, I believe that the many amateur musicians who play music at home for their own enjoyment, or play music in a community or school band, or sing in a choir, or play a rhythm instrument in a drum circle are providing themselves with a very powerful form of music therapy. They may benefit even more than some professional musicians who, for the sake of needing to make a living, may not often get to play their favorite type of music. For amateur musicians, this music therapy can go a long way toward reducing the stress built up from their day job, stimulating their creativity, and enhancing their joy of living.

If you have ever played a musical instrument, it's never too late to pick it up again. Maybe take a couple of lessons and join a community band, or "jam" with friends in your living room or garage, or sign up for a nighttime community-college band class, or join a church choir, or just get together with some friends and a guitar and sing.

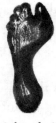

MORE MINDFUL MODES

Most of the practice of sitting meditation occurs during relatively brief practice periods. However, mindfulness is a much more pervasive form of meditation because it should ideally be practiced throughout much of our waking hours. The official website of the University of California at Los Angeles (UCLA) Mindful Awareness Research Center, which studies and teaches mindfulness, explains that mindfulness "invites us to stop, breathe, observe, and connect with one's inner experience. There are many ways to bring mindfulness into one's life, such as meditation, yoga, art, or time in nature."

What follows are some examples of how to incorporate the practice of mindfulness into some common activities of daily life.

MINDFULNESS OF EATING

Eating your food mindfully has several health benefits. First, enjoying the "taste of living" is a great way to appreciate the present moment. Second, when eating in the manner described below, you tend to make more healthy food choices. Chewing your food thoroughly and eating more slowly also helps your digestion. Lastly, when you eat mindfully, you usually consume less food, which helps prevent obesity.

To Eat Mindfully . . .

Focus your total attention on every aspect of eating your food. Savor the flavor, the texture, and the aroma of the food. Eat very slowly, chewing your food many times before swallowing. Try eating in silence for most of the meal. Don't eat and talk at the same time, or eat and talk and watch television at the same time. Simply enjoy the present moment, while focusing your awareness completely on eating.

I also recommend practicing the mealtime tradition of the monks and nuns of Deer Park and Plum Village monasteries, who begin every meal by first reciting what are called The Five Contemplations:

> This food is the gift of the whole universe—the earth, the sky,
> and much hard work.

May we eat in mindfulness so as to be worthy to receive it.

May we transform our unskillful states of mind and learn to eat in moderation.

May we take only foods that nourish us and prevent illness.

We accept this food to realize the path of understanding and love.

The Five Contemplations and many other mindful traditions practiced at the Deer Park and Plum Village monasteries can be found in the *Plum Village Chanting and Recitation Book*. These practices must prevent obesity because I note when I visit Deer Park Monastery that almost all the monks and nuns I see there are thin and energetic.

MINDFULNESS OF EXERCISING

Physical exercise can be a very healthy mindful activity. Walking meditation is a perfect example. More vigorous aerobic exercise can also work well as meditation. Elliptical exercise devices found at fitness centers provide a great low-impact aerobic workout. So does a stationary bicycle. These exercises may also be done while listening to music. Music then replaces the chanted mantra as a way to keep your mind from thinking. Pumping your arms and legs in time to the beat of the music feels great and helps pass the time while exercising.

In *The Inner Game of Tennis* (Random House, 1974), tennis pro W. Timothy Gallwey describes how being fully engaged in a vigorous sport like tennis can link your mind to your body in the present, reduce stress, and increase concentration and awareness of the here and now. This same mindful approach to exercise can be applied to almost any sport.

MINDFULNESS OF BEING WITH A PET

Mindfully spending time with a pet is a great opportunity to practice compassion and loving-kindness, as well as reduce stress. The companionship of a pet, such as a dog or a cat, can also reduce loneliness or "the blues," and enhance happiness.

Having a dog also helps take *you* on walks, which is good for both of you, physically and emotionally. I have two dogs: a white border collie named Bo, and a little red Aussie named Foxy. I know that when Bo, Foxy, and I go on a walk together, all three of us are happy. On those walks, it always intrigues me to notice how much pleasure other people we meet along the way get from talking to and petting my dogs.

People who frequently experience intermittent sadness or chronic loneliness might consider the benefits of what is called pet therapy. Pet therapy is now available at many hospitals and nursing homes. Petting a dog or cat can help people feel better. One medical research study showed that just petting a dog can lower a person's blood pressure. Another research study has shown that heart attack victims who have pets live longer.

MINDFULNESS OF DRIVING

When you were a kid, did you ever go to Disneyland and experience the thrill of driving your first car at the Disneyland Autopia? It was an exhilarating feeling to push your foot on the accelerator and command the steering wheel.

My other first driving experience came when I was ten years old and built a crude soap-box derby car with Radio Flyer wagon wheels for tires, a used refrigerator cardboard packing box for the chassis, a rope tied to the front axel to steer it, and a stick (and feet) to drag on the ground for brakes. It was such a feeling of adventure to go careening down from the top of the steeply curved street we kids called "the big banana."

But then something happens to the fun of driving for most of us after we grow up and own a real car. Despite the fact that the features of power, speed, steering, and brakes of even an inexpensive car are truly amazing, we tend to take them for granted. We drive like our minds are on auto-pilot—occupied with everything but driving: listening to the radio, talking, eating, thinking. When we get to where we are going, we don't remember anything that happened along the way. This is forgetfulness; the opposite of mindfulness.

When you practice mindfulness of driving it brings a lot of the youthful fun and adventure back into driving. Instead of being a stressful commute, driving can actually be a stress-reducing activity. While driving the car, smile and be aware of your in-breath and out-breath. Concentrate on the changing traffic patterns of cars streaming in front of you and around you. Open the window, smell the air, feel the temperature, and hear the wind and the sounds of the other cars just outside the skin of your vehicle. Enjoy the warp and woof of the city as you effortlessly pilot your amazing vehicle down the road.

Stay alert and alive to the present and *don't fall into a trance.* Avoid multitasking, like using the cell phone or eating while you drive. Turn off the radio and CD player. Try not to look at your watch. (You will get there when you get there.) Don't think about what you will be doing when you arrive at your destination.

When you see brake lights in front of you or a red traffic stoplight, don't get mad or frustrated. Regard these red lights as "bells of mindfulness" that serve to remind you to take three mindful breaths, not to hurry, and to just relax and enjoy the present moment.

Check out the musical-like rhythmic patterns that are created by driving past rows of trees, fence posts, telephone poles, and houses. While driving to work, I often feel that I'm in touch with the many rhythmic cycles of life: going to work and coming home, day and night, week to week, season to season, year to year. The rhythm of life is a groove.

MINDFULNESS OF SEX

You won't find mindfulness of sex discussed much by Zen Buddhist monks and nuns because they have taken a vow of celibacy. However, having sex with your loved one can be a wonderfully mindful experience.

Happily, my wife and I still have a healthy sex life. The stimulating, intimate joy of lovemaking is totally mindful. Focusing your entire attention on all the marvelous tactile sensations is a here-and-now delight. There are not only exciting tactile sensations in your fingers and genitals, but also the pleasures of caressing, pressing, squeezing, and massaging your lover with your arms, legs, and face—with your entire body. Your awareness is completely absorbed by the immediacy of the moment: the taste of kisses, the smell of the other's body, the rhythmic dance of the bodies intertwined. Perhaps there may be music playing in the background and the soft glow of candlelight. The opportunity to give pleasure and to satisfy the sexual desires of your partner is a manifestation of the love you share and your desire to help your partner be happy. The heightened energy of coming to a passionate climax is followed by the sweet release of tension. The orgasm triggers a release of endorphins, which bathe your brain, taking away all pain and slowing everything down in a seemingly timeless moment of complete repose and stillness.

MINDFULNESS AT WORK

For working people, many waking hours are spent at the workplace. Even when they have a job that they like, time spent at work can potentially be stressful, frustrating, tiring, or boring: that's why it's called work. Many people start the workday anticipating how nice it will be when the workday is over and they can go home, or how happy they will be when the work week is over and they can have fun on the weekend. This approach relegates the many hours of life at work to the status of being just unhappy "filler hours" sandwiched between more enjoyable hours when those people are off work.

However, if one wants to live a life filled with joy and happiness, it is necessary to extend the feeling of happiness into the workplace. To do this, avoid thinking about "your life at work" versus "your life not at work." As was discussed earlier in this chapter, if we take the view of the ultimate dimension of life, we can understand that all things are impermanent and transform, but they don't cease to exist—it is all one interconnected continuum. So, you can think of your life as a continuum, and that your entire life, even the time spent at work, can be spent practicing the path of joy, compassion, kindness, and peace.

At work, the best way to stay in this mode is to apply a mindful approach to the workday. This doesn't mean that you don't do any thinking at work—as most jobs require thinking to accomplish the task at hand. Here mindfulness means that you stay fully engaged in each task you do at work. Don't rush. Don't allow your mind to jump ahead to anticipate all the appointments and tasks that await you later in the day. Instead, take each encounter or appointment one at a time, while you stay *in the moment.*

Adopting this approach to working really starts the night before. You need to get to sleep early enough to wake up early in the morning, feeling refreshed, with enough time that you don't have to rush to get ready for work. (See the section "Beginning Anew" on page 168.) From the beginning of your day practice mindfulness while bathing, getting dressed, eating breakfast, or while sipping tea or coffee.

While doing these simple morning tasks, I focus on my breathing. Sometimes I also silently repeat two of the pairs of guidewords used in Buddha's Breathing Exercises for several minutes. Those two key pairs of guidewords are "calm/ease" and "smile/release." During my in-breath, I silently say the word "calm," which reminds me to slow down and go back to the calm center, or island, within myself. During my out-breath I say the word "ease," which reminds me to ease my muscles and thereby prevent them from tightening up as I get ready for the workday. During the few minutes it takes to get dressed, instead of going through a whole-body scan while easing each body part one at a time, I may ease the entire core of my body all at once. And with each out-breath I can feel my entire body core—including my face, throat, chest, and abdomen—relax all together.

Then, after a couple of minutes, I move on to "smile/release." Saying "smile" during my in-breath reminds me to lighten up my face by smiling with my lips, eyes, and eyebrows. On the next out-breath, saying "release" reminds me to release any negative feelings—such as anxiety, fear, jealousy, anger, sadness, or frustration—and also to release the tendency to always be thinking and obsessively planning for my day ahead.

If you take this approach, instead of anxiously anticipating the stress of the day ahead, you start the day in a good mood and can look forward to your encounters at work as opportunities to practice kindness and compassion. Approaching the job with kindness and compassion toward people with whom you interact at work will enhance your own happiness. Be thankful that you have a job to go to, where there are tasks and people who will benefit from your time and attention. If you had no job to do or responsibilities to fulfill, life would be rather boring, and it would be difficult to earn an adequate income.

When you get to work, smile when you see your coworkers. They are impermanent, they won't always be there. Appreciate that they are there today and are willing to help handle the workload; and, therefore, they are closely interconnected with you. Cherish your coworkers and treat them with kindness, compassion, and respect. Don't rush past them. Stop and talk with them, and take a sincere interest in their sufferings and aspirations.

At work, when negative feelings arise in you, it is important to embrace and take good care of those negative feelings. Do this by taking the time to recognize the negative feeling and breathe with it, in order to reduce and transform any anger, disappointment, frustration, or sadness. Return to your calm center frequently throughout your workday—maybe for just two or three mindful breaths at a time—which enables you to see that your negative emotions are just transient reactions in the ultimate dimension. Practicing walking meditation at lunchtime can also help calm your negative feelings and transform anger or sadness.

As the workday proceeds, don't frantically rush to get the day's work done and "clear your in-box." Remember that when you finally die, there will still be stuff left in your in-box. Just take your time to be fully mindful of each task, without worrying that it is slowing you down or that it is just something to get through before the "real action" can happen.

And try not to try too hard, because as James Taylor sings in his song "Secret O' Life," life is "just a lovely ride." This is your life, here and now; it's not a rehearsal. Don't put off your happiness until later—find joy in the present moment right now and across the continuum of your life.

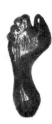

MEDITATIONS FOR A GOOD NIGHT'S SLEEP

Here are three meditation techniques you can use to treat insomnia.

1. **If you can't fall asleep, or if you wake up in the middle of the night and can't get back to sleep.** While lying in bed, use AH-OM Breath meditation described in Chapter 1 to help you fall asleep naturally. It works better than counting sheep.

2. **If your mind is agitated and full of thoughts that prevent you from falling to sleep.** Instead of using the AH-OM mantra, try the meditation method that follows:

   • "Breathing in, I am aware my mind is full of thoughts. Breathing out, my mind is becoming like still water." Repeat this while concentrating on your in-breath and out-breath.

   • After a few minutes, transition to simply saying these two guide-words: "deep/still." The word "deep" reminds you to concentrate on taking a deep, full in-breath. During your out-breath, silently say the word "still" and imagine your mind becoming as still as a large, placid lake. This doesn't work instantly, but after ten to twenty minutes you will probably fall asleep and wake up feeling refreshed.

3. **Lastly, here is another meditation variation I occasionally use if I awaken in the middle of the night and can't get back to sleep.** I get out of bed and sit in a comfortable recliner chair with my head, back, arms, and legs supported by the pads of the chair and a soft blanket drawn over my body. Then I start the AH-OM Breath meditation and combine it with a body scan meditation as follows below.

   • I breathe in through my nose while silently saying "AHHHH," concentrating on my in-breath, all the way through.

   • I silently say "OMMMM" during the out-breath. I try to feel as if I were able to breathe out through an imaginary hole in part of the body, as I focus on each body part, one at a time—including forehead, jaw, tongue, arms, fingers, back, chest, abdomen, pelvic sphincters, buttocks, legs and toes—for about three breaths each. With each out-breath the muscles of the body become progressively more relaxed.

- If I am still awake at the end of the sequence above, I might start silently saying the "deep/still" mantra along with my in-breath and out-breath. After a while, I will usually fall asleep. Even if I don't, after forty-five minutes of this, my mind and body feel totally restored and ready to get up and start my morning. It might then only be 4:30 or 5:00 A.M., which gives me some time to work on a creative project before I slowly and mindfully start the rest of the morning activities while getting ready to go to work.

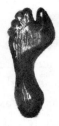

THE STRESS RELIEVER PHYSICIANS CAN TEACH IN THEIR OFFICE

Patients can be taught to meditate by doctors who have a busy office practice. But this is difficult to do within the time frame of a typical office visit. In order to acquaint patients with what meditation is, I have free handouts of articles about meditation in my waiting room for patients to take home and read. I also have printed handouts of recommended books, audiotapes, and CDs patients may purchase at local bookstores or online to learn about meditation at home.

Furthermore, when seeing patients with medical complaints in the office, I may identify people who have stress-induced symptoms or other illnesses who would obviously benefit from the practice of meditation. They are invited to come to a group meditation class that meets in the waiting room of my office for an hour in the early evening, once a week for a few weeks. I teach a series of these meditation classes every three or four months. People can easily learn the basic meditation technique in two lessons. But each new group of students usually comes to several classes in order to learn some alternate meditation exercises, a little about the Zen perspective, and how the practice of meditation can be incorporated into the normal activities of daily life.

When a patient's main problem is how to cope with anxiety and stress, I do have the time within the confines of a typical office visit to teach the following meditation breathing exercise. It is called The Stress Reliever (an abbreviated version of Buddha's Breathing Exercises). In a few minutes, I can review the basics of how to do the meditation exercise with my patient. Then I ask him or her to practice it at home on a daily basis and see if it helps reduce their anxiety and stress. I also give them a printed copy of the exercise, as shown below, to help my patients remember the instructions later.

THE STRESS RELIEVER

Try to spend less time regretting what has happened in the past, or worrying about and fearing what might happen in the future. A method to help you focus attention on the present is to concentrate on your breath. Doing this quickly links your mind to your body in the present.

Try doing the breathing exercises described below for ten to fifteen minutes once or twice a day. These exercises can effectively be done either while sitting in a chair or while lying down in bed. Start by directing your attention to your breath. Continue to be aware of your in-breath and out-breath while silently saying to yourself these three pairs of guidewords:

1. **In/Out:** Silently say the word "in" on your in-breath, and focus your mind on your in-breath all the way through (not just at the beginning of inhalation). Feel all the sensations of air coming in through your nose and filling up your lungs as you notice your chest and abdomen expand. Silently say to yourself the word "out" during your out-breath. Feel all the sensations associated with breathing out, and stay concentrated on it all the way through to the end of your out-breath. Do this for a couple of minutes, then go on to the next pair of guidewords.

2. **Deep/Slow:** Continue to follow your breath. During your in-breath say to yourself the word "deep." During your out-breath say the word

"slow." Upon doing this, you will notice your breath naturally becomes more deep and slow, more pleasant, relaxing, and cleansing. After a couple of minutes go on to the last pair of guidewords.

3. **Calm/Ease:** Silently say the word "calm" during your in-breath. This signifies calming your mind, so it becomes more peaceful, still, and centered. Say the word "ease" during your out-breath. This means to ease and relax the muscles of the body. (You are now going beyond linking the mind to the breath, and beginning to link your mind to your entire body. This allows the mind and body to relax and heal the stress.) It is often helpful, while saying the word "ease," to mentally perform a complete body scan. First, focus your attention on the top of the head and forehead muscles as you feel those muscles relax. Then, with successive breaths, progressively relax muscles of the face, jaw and tongue, neck and shoulders, arms and hands, upper and lower back, chest and abdomen, legs and feet. Spend more time on any part of the body that is painful, stiff, or tight.

Here are some other stress-reducing suggestions: Pay attention to healing elements around you—such as the blue sky and the green grass and trees, the sound of birds and the smell of flowers, the calming effect of the ocean, mountains, lakes, and streams, and your ability to walk and exercise. Let your friends and family nourish you by their concern and touch. Don't withdraw from them thinking, "I can handle this stress on my own." Try to let go of grudges, egotistical pride, and frustration with other people for not being perfect.

MORE MEDITATIONS AND HEALING PRACTICES

Please take a look at the Mindfulness Bibliography at the end of this book for a list of books and audio CDs containing additional meditation methods. If you prefer to close your eyes and be guided through several of the meditations that were included in this chapter, listen to the *Teaching Meditation* audio CD that accompanies this book.

CHAPTER FIVE

Advanced Meditation Concepts for Deepening Your Practice

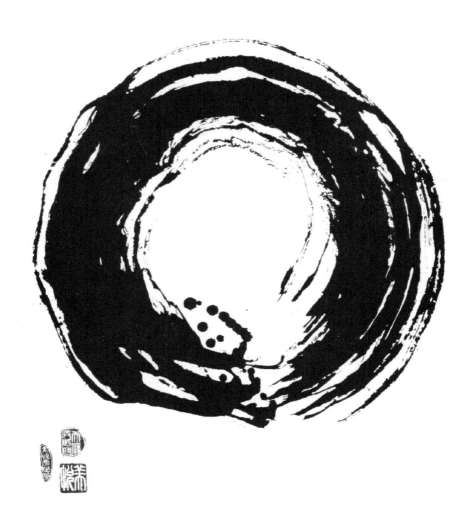

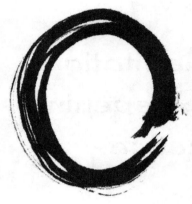

This chapter on advanced meditation concepts presents a unified approach to the practice of meditation, rather than simply seeing the process as a menu of optional meditation exercises that you choose from in some haphazard way. It focuses on how to transform the negative feelings and states of mind, which can create obstacles in your meditative efforts and keep you from experiencing its deeper benefits, into positive ones. This chapter more fully explores Zen concepts concerning happiness, love, self, community (sangha), the role of thinking in our lives, and the notion of aimlessness. Also explained is how to correct previous unskillful behavior by making a fresh start or "beginning anew," and the benefit of viewing life from the perspective of "the ultimate dimension."

THE PRACTICE

"The practice" refers to the practice of meditation in the context of a life of wisdom and morality. It's called "the practice" because you have to practice it regularly for it to help, and with regular practice you get better at it. However, you never get it 100 percent right for long. This section provides a unified overview of how the practice works in real-life situations, and discusses aids and obstacles to the practice of meditation.

TRANSFORM NEGATIVE FEELINGS

Negative states of mind occur from time to time in everybody. The negative states might be feelings of distress, frustration, anger, anxiety, sorrow, fear, boredom, depression, or feeling rushed or ignored.

Throughout your daily life, whenever you notice the presence of a negative mental state, practice meditation to understand the roots of your negative feeling, and to transform it into a more positive state of mind. So, practice these meditation techniques any time of day or night, not just during preplanned formal meditation sessions. You may not always have the time to start a formal meditation exercise immediately. But as soon as you notice a negative feeling or thought, taking just three mindful breaths (or AH-OM breaths) can be enough to enable you to center your mind and body, and restore your sense of calm and joy. Later, you can practice concentrated sitting or walking meditation to gain more insight into the roots of your negative feeling.

As part of the practice, you become a compassionate "witness" to the emotional states inside of yourself. Ram Dass, in *Be Here Now*, calls it a process of "calming, centering, centering, calming, extricating [yourself] from the drama . . . You're standing on a bridge watching yourself go by. Wow! Look at that!"

But, you are not just a passive observer. In *Full Catastrophe Living*, Jon Kabat-Zinn writes, "It would be incorrect to think of meditation as a passive process. It takes a good deal of energy and effort to regulate your attention and to remain genuinely calm and non-reactive. But, paradoxically, mindfulness does not involve trying to get anywhere or feel anything special. Rather it involves allowing yourself to be where you already are, to become more familiar with your own actual experience moment by moment."

EMBRACE

The practice is to first *recognize* your negative feeling. Then, after you are fully aware of the negative feeling, you use meditation to "embrace" and calm it. At the 2006 spring retreat in Plum Village, Thich Nhat Hanh explained, "Embracing means not to suppress or fight it [the negative feeling], but to deal with it in the most nonviolent, gentle way. Like a mother who tenderly holds her ailing baby, there is solidarity, there is support, there is care. The mother transfers her energy of gentleness and love to the baby, so the baby suffers less. That is not simply observation, but participation."

However, meditation takes time to do its work. "Embracing" a negative feeling doesn't reduce the suffering immediately. It's like cooking potatoes; if you take them out of the boiling water after two minutes, they are not ready to eat. You must leave them in longer to complete the cooking.

When you are under stress at work, or your personal life is plagued with frustration, anger, sadness, fear, or physical illness, you might feel like you don't have time for things like meditation. But, this is when you *most* need to make the time for the healing power of meditation to help you overcome these difficulties.

LOOKING DEEPLY

Meditation enables you to attain a calm, clear state of mind. Then, as you continue to meditate, insights about your negative feeling may spring into your awareness. This is what is called "looking deeply" into the root causes of the negative feeling.

It is not enough to just use meditation to feel calm and peaceful. You must also be willing to take the next step and concentrate your mind in meditation in order to look deeply into the root causes of difficult emotions like anger and fear. You must be willing to use meditation to skillfully "lock into battle" with these negative feelings, though it may take a concentrated effort over days of work to fully deal with them.

To facilitate this process, it helps to remind yourself to let go of jealousy, greed, intolerance, past grudges, hatred, and fear. We also enhance our ability to generate insight when we are constantly mindful of the wisdom of impermanence, interconnectedness, nonattachment, and compassion. So, if I am trying to look deeply into a negative feeling or problem, right before sitting meditation I might go over a mental checklist of these core principles and focus on how they might apply to the specific situation at hand. Or I might recite a poem or gatha that contains key guidewords (see examples on pages 189 and 190), in order to help trigger insight during a later meditation practice.

WATERING THE SEEDS

Zen teachings refer to so-called seeds, which normally lie dormant in the mind in what is called the store consciousness. These seeds represent standard behaviors and associated emotions that occur in us as we react to a variety of situations. When these seeds come into our awareness, they are said to have manifested in our mind consciousness. At this point, they are called mental formations. This is a lot like having many programs stored in the memory of your personal computer. At any time you might click open a particular program, which then manifests onto the desktop of your computer so you can work with it.

Thich Nhat Hanh compares your mind consciousness to a living room where you receive guests. Some are unpleasant guests, who, due to circumstances force their way into your living room and you must deal with them. These unpleasant guests are the manifestation of negative seeds like anger, fear, sorrow, jealousy, greed, hatred, and intolerance.

Practicing meditation promotes the manifestation of positive mental formations, also called "watering the good seeds." Examples of positive mental formations include happiness, loving-kindness, freshness, energy, compassion, mindfulness, concentration, nondiscrimination, humor, and liberation. Thich Nhat Hanh explains these positive mental formations are like very pleasant guests that you can invite into your living room. And the key point is this: spending more time with pleasant guests in the living room of your mind leaves less time to be with those unpleasant guests!

So the practice of meditation and other skillful means is to not only skillfully deal with negative mental formations, but also to actively encourage the manifestation of positive seeds.

This conceptual process is very similar to what were, at the time, radical ideas proposed by Baruch Spinoza, a seventeenth-century Dutch philosopher of Portuguese Jewish origin. In *Looking for Spinoza: Joy, Sorrow, and the Feeling Brain* (Harvest Books, 2003), neuroscientist Antonio Damasio explains, "Spinoza asks the individual to attempt a break between the emotionally competent stimuli that can trigger negative emotions—passions such as fear, anger, jealousy, sadness—and the very mechanisms that enact emotion. Instead, the individual should substitute emotionally competent stimuli capable of triggering positive, nourishing emotions." Meditation enables us to achieve this.

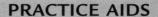

PRACTICE AIDS

In Chapter 3 we discussed the path to enlightenment. Here we will explore the seven conditions, identified by Buddha, that help facilitate progress on the path to enlightenment. He called them the Seven Factors of Enlightenment. In addition to mindfulness, they include: investigation of reality (curiosity), energy, happiness, tranquility, concentration, and equanimity.

CURIOSITY AND ENERGY

Having the curiosity and energy to investigate reality are prerequisites to making progress on the path. This is not passive practice but an active investigation of what is happening in the present using practices such as meditation that are designed to actively transform negative states.

Albert Einstein called many of his investigations of reality "thought experiments." Similarly, I consider meditations to be "mind experiments." (Not *thought* experiments, because during meditation thinking is minimized and awareness of the present is maximized.) It takes curiosity to investigate what might result from meditation-mind experiments such as Pebble Meditation or Meditation on the Whole Person, which were described in Chapter 4.

HAPPINESS AND TRANQUILITY

If we stay mindful of the many natural elements within us and around us, they can contribute much to our happiness and tranquility. Our ability to walk and smile, be aware of our breath, the blue sky, the green grass and trees, the fragrance of flowers, the refreshing feel of a cool summer breeze, the warmth of the sun, the mystery of the moon and the stars, the beauty of the ocean, lakes, and streams, the sweet taste of fresh fruit, the singing of birds and the sound of laughter: these are a few of the precious things that permeate our lives and can contribute to our happiness.

CONCENTRATION

Concentration takes practice. The more we practice, the better our concentration becomes. The more deeply we stay concentrated in meditation, the more we can then realize valuable insights about our life.

EQUANIMITY

Equanimity has more than one meaning in Zen Buddhism. It means to feel calm and centered, with inner peace. It also means to act unselfishly, with equal treatment for all living things, and without hostility or ill will.

PRACTICE OBSTACLES

In *A Path with Heart,* psychologist and former Buddhist monk Jack Kornfield describes the obstacles he encountered when trying to apply Buddhist teachings he had learned to his normal life. Kornfield writes, "My first ten years of systematic spiritual practice were conducted primarily through my mind . . . I developed concentration . . . I had visions, revelations, and a variety of deep awakenings." But later, when Kornfield returned to the United States after years of practicing in Asian monasteries, he still had a lot of frustration in dealing with people in his normal life. He was then "forced to shift my whole practice . . . from the mind to the heart. I began a long and difficult process of reclaiming my emotions . . . of learning how to feel my feelings, and what to do with the powerful forces of human connection."

Kornfield came also to recognize the importance of his own body in this process. He adds, "After ten years of focusing on emotional work, I realized I had neglected my body . . . The way I treat my body is not disconnected from the way I treat my family . . . The vision of my practice has expanded to include, not just my own body or heart, but all of life, the relationships we hold, and the environment that sustains us."

As Kornfield discovered, consistently following "the practice" is not always easy as there are some common obstacles to overcome along the path. Buddha described five obstacles, or impediments, that interfere with the practice of meditation. The obstacles are torpor (laziness), restlessness, anger, regret, and doubt.

For me, the first three obstacles are the most challenging. To overcome laziness and restlessness, it helps to remind myself of the Dharma wisdom by reading books, reciting spiritual poems, and sharing experiences with friends on the path of awakening.

Anger still remains an obstacle for me. It often rears its ugly head just when I least expect it. Buddha described this phenomenon metaphorically in his famous discourse (sermon) called the Lotus Sutra. Buddha taught that the eye and the ear are like an ocean. Buddha said that a person might be feeling good one minute, metaphorically floating serenely on a raft on the surface of the ocean. Then, the next minute, they might see or hear something that causes their peacefully floating raft to quickly become swamped and capsized by "heaving waves and undersea monsters" of raging anger, fear, or despair. But, if that person can skillfully use meditation to take care of their negative emotional reactions, they can reduce their suffering and avoid becoming drowned in anger, fear, and despair.

Regret takes care of itself if you keep your mind focused on the present, instead of remaining mired in thoughts about the past. Doubt is not a problem when you begin to notice for yourself the positive effects meditation is having on your life.

 ## VALIDATION OF THE PRACTICE

In the book *The Open Road: The Global Journey of the Fourteenth Dalai Lama* (Alfred A. Knopf, 2008), author Pico Iyer states that "Siddhartha Gautama, the Buddha, was first and foremost an empiricist, a scientist of self." In Iyer's book, the Buddha is also likened to a doctor who asks his patient to judge the validity of his advice by the results that are produced.

The Buddha knew that no teaching is the perfect absolute truth for all time, and he did not ask his students to accept his teaching on unconditional blind faith. Instead, Buddha invited each person to verify the teaching for his or herself. In *Old Path White Clouds,* Thich Nhat Hanh reports that Buddha was to have said, "Believe and accept only those things which accord with your reason . . . and those things which in practice bring benefit and happiness to yourselves and others." And, in the last days of his life, he rejected the idea of passing the mantle of leadership of his sangha to another person, but instead Siddhartha told his disciples, "Every person should be a lamp unto himself."

So, what is the best way to validate or verify that the practice of wisdom, morality, and meditation can help one achieve a healthier, happier, and more enlightened life? Echoing the Buddha, I would put it this way: Don't believe in the validity of the Zen perspective just because it sounds logical or presents a vision of a grand scheme of life. Instead, validation comes from the practice itself and the positive way it affects your life path.

PRACTICE PEARLS

In this last section, topics like sustaining happiness, true love, emptiness of self, community, and the role of thinking are further clarified to see how they fit into the practice of wisdom, morality, and meditation. Also, the concepts of aimlessness, beginning anew, and the ultimate dimension are defined.

SUSTAINING HAPPINESS

One of the main purposes of life is to seek happiness. But what type of happiness? Zen teaches that there are qualitatively different forms of happiness. For instance, Zen discourages happiness derived from inflicting suffering on another person. You might find some temporary satisfaction from getting revenge against a perceived enemy. But this is not the type of happiness we should be seeking. Experience shows that harbor-

ing grudges and acting out of hatred ultimately tears down our happiness and leaves us feeling agitated and angry. Also, the enemy you best-
ed, or their supporters, will eventually find a way to get back at you,
perpetuating cycles of revenge and unhappiness.

Simple, natural pleasures—like the fragrant smell of fresh flowers or
the warm touch of a friend—can make us happy. But the happiness does-
n't last forever. So, Zen teachings place a high value on the feeling of
freedom that comes from the practice of nonattachment. We might be
happy enjoying the beauty of nature or time spent with a friend. However, if we also understand the natural order of impermanence, then we
don't get caught in despair when separation inevitably occurs. Therefore,
it is the deep appreciation of natural pleasures that we can encounter
every day, tempered by the wisdom of nonattachment, that can sustain
our sense of joy over a lifetime.

In addition to distinguishing between qualitatively different types of
happiness, Siddhartha Gautama taught that there are also relative degrees
of suffering. For example, he taught that people suffer endlessly when
they cling to gratification of their own sense pleasures. On the other
hand, if you are unsuccessful in trying to help someone you care about,
that may also cause you some sadness and suffering. However, Siddhartha
stated that people suffer much less when their suffering is born of com-
passionately trying to help another person.

Happiness is not only healthy for you, as research shows (see Chapter 2), but your happiness also has positive effects on the people around
you. For example, the most precious gift parents can give their children
is to be happy themselves. This is because when children see that their
parents are happy and loving, this gives the children a feeling of happiness, peace, and a sense of optimism. Conversely, when children see
that their parents are fighting and unhappy, it is very difficult for the
children to develop a sense of happiness and security. This is not only
true of children. Because we are interconnected with all other people,
our happiness has a positive effect on their emotional state as well.

Sustaining happiness requires the following important practices:

- Organize your day to allow the seeds of joy and happiness to be frequently watered every day. The regular practice of meditation helps

to water the seeds of happiness. Also, as much as possible, dwell in the wonders of the present by taking the time to mindfully appreciate the natural healing elements around you, like the blue sky, the green grass, the fresh air, the fragrance of flowers, and other simple pleasures that promote a positive joyful energy to manifest in the mind. For example, I often take walks by the ocean. For me, it is spiritually uplifting to experience the sound of the ocean's crashing waves and the sight of its vast power and beauty. The ocean has the reassuring yet mysterious quality of remaining the same while, at the same time, constantly changing. This can serve as a metaphor for our life.

- A happy person must also be able to let go of hate, anger, and fear, and have the capacity to forgive mistakes in other people.

- Be a nonjudgmental, compassionate witness to your own life. Regardless of temporary setbacks and disappointments, learn to accept "what is" without anger or sadness. And if you need to take action to change something, do so without negativity.

- Actively encourage within yourself the seeds of love and compassion. By practicing loving speech and compassionate listening you will become more pleasant and fresh.

- Happiness is increased by maintaining nourishing relationships with your family members and a few close friends.

- Happiness requires reasonable health. So, pay attention to the health needs of your body, including getting proper exercise, rest, nutrition, and medical care.

Sustaining happiness in a world full of suffering is truly an art. Like a musician practicing his instrument every day, regularly practicing the skills mentioned above will bring about a harmonious happiness in the here and now. Don't expect your happiness to occur at some future time after you have achieved some personal goal, or be waiting to achieve happiness in some distant afterlife. Happiness is now or never.

TRUE LOVE

Buddha had much to say about what constitutes true love. In *Old Path White Clouds,* Thich Nhat Hanh describes Buddha as saying, "If our love is based on a selfish desire to possess others, our love will make them feel trapped. Gradually the love between us will turn to anger and hatred."

Buddha went on to say, "Love is understanding . . . If you want your loved ones to be happy, you must learn to understand their sufferings and their aspirations. When you understand, you will then know how to relieve their sufferings and how to help them fulfill their aspirations. That is true love."

You might ask your spouse, child, parent, or other loved one, "Do you think I sufficiently understand your suffering and your aspirations?" If the answer is no, that you don't understand, ask them to help you. Then listen very deeply to what they say. Out of that understanding, you will know what to do, or what not to do, to help bring them happiness.

At a 2007 retreat at Deer Park Monastery, Thich Nhat Hanh described the four main elements of true love as taught by Buddha:

- **Offer your beloved compassion.** Compassion is the desire to want to understand him or her, and the desire to relieve their suffering. Sustaining compassion over time requires having the capacity to forgive imperfections in your partner. It helps to understand that after people grow up, they still harbor many of the fears and insecurities they acquired when they were children. So, you might try to increase your "eyes of compassion" by looking at your grown-up child, your parent, or your lover as if he or she were still a five-year-old child—wounded, vulnerable, and suffering. You will then be more forgiving of their apparent flaws and mistakes.

- **Treat the other person with kindness.** Kindness is defined as actions you take that reduce suffering and/or enhance happiness in another person. However, in order to bring loving-kindness to another person, you must first learn to be kind to yourself. Develop loving-kindness toward yourself by nourishing your qualities of freshness, solidity, calmness, space, and freedom. (*Pebble Meditation* on page 118 can help you do this.) You can then offer to your beloved that freshness, solidity, calmness, space, and freedom, coupled with acts of kindness, that will help him or her to be happy, too.

- **Bring to your beloved and yourself a sense of joy.** Look and see if enough joy is there. If enough joy is not there, then you should do something (or stop doing something) in order to frequently water the seeds of gladness and happiness in yourself. You might do this by mindful walking and breathing (see walking meditation on page 105 and Buddha's Breathing Exercises on page 114). You must also develop the capacity to "let go." Let go of anger, grudges, and fears. Let go of thinking that your happiness requires achieving some external goal like a more highly paid job, an advanced degree, a big house, an expensive car, or successfully completing all your projects. You need the courage to let go of some of these things in order to have more space and freedom to be happy. You can then bring that sense of happiness and joy to your loved one.

- **Equanimity.** Equanimity is inclusive, nondiscriminatory, nonjudgmental, and peaceful. Leave no frontiers between yourself and the other person, and include everyone in your love.

For love to stay alive, it is necessary to nourish your love every day with the four elements listed above. Try to bring compassion, kindness, joy, and forgiveness to your relationship *each day* so your love can be watered and nourished. Without constant watering, your love will soon die and turn to hatred. Once love has died we cannot be happy. You must use deep listening and loving speech to revive love that is dead or dying. In true love there is no pride. The other person's suffering is your suffering. So look at your husband/wife/partner, your son/daughter, or your mother/father and ask yourself again, Have I sufficiently tried to truly understand their suffering and their aspirations? Then offer your loved ones compassion and kindness to help relieve their suffering. It is just as important to take the time to listen deeply to their hopes and dreams in order to find ways to help them attain their aspirations.

EMPTINESS OF SELF

Zen's concept of "the self" is subtle and can be tricky to understand, especially when it comes to the somewhat confusing phrase "emptiness of self." As discussed earlier, Buddha taught that what we normally call "the self" or "the person" can be divided into five separate components: the body, feelings, perceptions, mental formations, and consciousness. All these components are constantly changing (impermanent), and are constantly being affected by a multitude of enabling conditions (interdependent). Each component within a person, therefore, is said to be "empty" of a permanent, separate existence. The basic meaning of emptiness is as follows: This is, because that is. And nothing is permanent.

Since all things are interdependent and impermanent, this property called "emptiness" affects everything. This concept is called the "emptiness of all dharmas." The word "dharma" in Buddhism has two primary meanings. When capitalized, Dharma usually refers to the teachings of Buddha. On the other hand, the term dharma (not capitalized) means all the constituent factors of the experienced world—including all mental and physical phenomena. Buddha taught that all dharmas are empty. The Buddha went on to explain, "If we say that all dharmas are empty, what are they empty of? . . . The emptiness of all dharmas refers to the fact that all dharmas are empty of a permanent and unchanging self. That is the meaning of the emptiness of all dharmas . . . Empty means empty of self."

But, even though all things, including people, are empty of self, they do exist. A glass may appear to be empty, but it is also full of air. Similarly, everything is empty, but at the same time everything is full of the cosmos. A rose, for example, may appear to be a separate entity, but it is completely made of, and dependent on, many non-rose elements for its existence—like the rain, the sun, the soil, the seed, the farmer, the farmer's ancestors, time, space, and so on. Buddha described it most simply this way: "The source of one thing is all things." In 1798, a similar sentiment was expressed by the English romantic poet William Wordsworth. In his poem "Tintern Abbey" he wrote, "For nature then . . . to me was all in all."

Like the rose, we humans are also dependent on a multitude of enabling conditions for our existence. But while we do exist, we are also not permanent unchanging entities. Buddhists see the self as like a river. A river may appear to exist as an enduring entity; however, the water within the river is actually constantly changing. Despite the fact that we seem to be an enduring entity, our body and mind are also constantly changing.

But, despite this lack of permanence, we do have a sense of continuity of self. I would argue that the feeling of continuity of self is due to the interdependent nature of our lives, where one thing leads to another as a consequence of various preceding causes and conditions.

David Galin, a neuropsychologist at the University of California, San Francisco, proposes that, over time, we manifest a multitude of selves. Dr. Galin writes, "It is readily apparent that a person, like any complex system, might be capable of different patterns of organization (selves) . . . I propose that we explicitly designate that 'person' is extended over time, and 'self' is the current organization of the person." This formulation is similar to the German novelist Hermann Hesse's poetic description of a person being composed of multiple selves, with the pieces of their personality frequently changing and reorganizing over time. Hesse wrote about this concept in his novel *Steppenwolf* (see Chapter 6).

Mark Epstein, a psychotherapist with a Buddhist perspective, talks about a constantly changing ego arising within the self. In an interview for Amazon.com, Epstein explains,

I think the ego arises and disappears thousands of times during the day, within that true nature of the self. So I think it's a mistake to see the ego as the embodiment of the true nature, but it's also a mistake to see the ego as not existing at all. We all need egos in order to carry out our business, but what Buddhism says, and what I think is true, is that we're all much too identified with those egos, and we're trying to keep them pumped up all the time, instead of realizing that the ego, like everything else, is arising and passing away moment to moment, and it has no inherent reality.

The above descriptions about what constitutes the self are themselves impermanent and eventually also will change. That is the nature of all dharmas. It is, however, interesting to read many new Western-based authors emerging to add their voices to the discussion about how the Zen perspective, including the concept of self, applies to our lives today. The phenomenon of a developing tradition of a Western-oriented Buddhism is the theme of Joseph Goldstein's book *One Dharma: The Emerging Western Buddhism* (HarperCollins, 2002). It is wonderful to see Buddha's original ideas being further developed and adapted over time as the Dharma is applied to the American experience.

SANGHA (COMMUNITY)

Sangha means "community" in Sanskrit. The people in a community provide vital support for one another on many interconnected levels. For Buddhists, sangha usually refers to their practice community. But most of us have several sanghas to which we belong. One sangha is your family. You share a common genetic heritage and history that uniquely binds you together for life. This group includes all your ancestors. You would not be here without them.

The Zen monks and nuns at Deer Park Monastery also venerate two other groups of ancestors: land ancestors and spiritual ancestors. Land ancestors are the people who preceded you in owning and having responsibility for stewardship of the land on which you live and work and play. This sangha reminds you of how you are connected to the environment and the people who have preceded you here. This group includes your neighbors with whom you share the land. It is important to be empathetic, considerate, and supportive of the other people in the neighborhood.

The third group of ancestors is your spiritual ancestors. This important sangha deserves much respect. We honor these ancestors by reading and studying their ideas, and trying to apply their collective wisdom to our life path. This sangha includes your practice community, the people who reinforce your practice. All practitioners can benefit from this type of spiritual interconnectedness.

Another sangha that plays an important role in our lives is the community of people with whom we work. The quality of the relationships we have with the women and men at our workplace makes a big difference to the amount of stress or happiness we feel in our lives. We should make every effort to get along with our coworkers and treat them with kindness and compassion.

Other work-related sanghas are the professional organizations to which you may belong. In my case, this includes the medical staff of my hospital and the greater medical community. It is quite clear that I could not do what I do professionally without the support of my medical colleagues. Before I learned to deeply respect the interconnectedness of the sangha, I used to get very bored at medical staff meetings. But now I understand that just by being at these meetings, I lend my support to the group in an important way—even if I say nothing during the entire meeting. Once I understood this, it took the pressure off me to come up with some words of wisdom to contribute to the meeting in order to justify my taking the time to attend. Now, when I go to the meetings of my medical sangha, I usually just smile and breathe, and I'm not bored.

THINKING

In order to meditate, it is necessary to suppress the normal thinking process. This is not meant to imply that thinking is bad or always to be avoided. On the contrary, to be able to think is good. We need thinking to survive and thrive. As a doctor, I must use the thinking process to diagnose and treat patients. The formulation of a medical treatment plan requires a thought process that involves planning for the future and taking into account past experience. It is also necessary for people to have thoughts and language in order to become consciously aware of certain important insights, and to store those insights in one's memory for future use. Thinking is obviously an important and necessary element of life.

However, it is not necessary for people to generate thought processes in order to tap into their intuitive wisdom. It is also not necessary to think to simply be in touch with the wonders of the present, which can promote positive states of mind. As important as thinking is, we must remember that we are far more than a thinking mind. Meditating is one way to avoid becoming trapped by the "tyranny of the thinking mind," which often dominates our awareness.

I have a very good friend who asked me how I reconcile the present-oriented, peaceful practice of mindfulness with the need to give medical orders and do the other directive, multitasking things doctors do throughout the day. The answer is that you have to learn to skillfully shift back and forth between normal consciousness and mindfulness consciousness, while trying to remain unhurried and totally focused on the task at hand. That takes practice, and we don't get the practice right all the time. However, as time goes on, I am able to spend a larger percentage of my workday in mindfulness; but it will never be 100 percent. For most of us, the workday is a constant dance, shifting between thinking and doing and being.

AIMLESSNESS

Aimlessness is a state of being where you don't put any thing, or any goal, in front of yourself and aim for it. Aimlessness is an understanding that what you are looking for is already there. You are wonderful just as you are in the present moment. It is the Zen concept of arriving at the beginning.

Don't strive or aim for enlightenment, because there is no way to enlightenment—enlightenment is the way. Similarly, there is no way to peace—peace is the way. There is no way to happiness—happiness is the way. Happiness is then possible throughout the day when you breathe, eat, or walk.

Aimlessness is a door to liberation. You can step through that door at any time. Then peace is every step.

BEGINNING ANEW

The phrase "beginning anew" refers to the opportunity we always have to put the past behind us and start fresh all over again.

After two people have looked deeply into the cause of interpersonal anger or frustration, understanding that nobody is perfect, they can then agree to forgive each other and begin anew in friendship, compassion, kindness, and love.

Similarly, you should also forgive yourself for not being a perfect practitioner of meditation and having at times acted unskillfully. For example, sometimes I unskillfully act out of anger or frustration, or allow bad habits to creep into my daily activities, such as overeating or permitting too much multitasking and work pressures to get the best of me.

Nevertheless, every day brings an opportunity to begin anew as a practitioner of mindfulness. When you wake up in the morning, smile and tell yourself that you have twenty-four more hours to live in this wonderful world. If you still live with other family members or pets, you can hug your spouse and children and pet the dog or cat, and be happy they are still there sharing your life. You can also be happy that it is so convenient to roll out of bed and just twist a little knob and out pours clean water with which to bathe yourself. The feel of bathing can be such a wonderful, cleansing, mindful experience. Don't rush, or start thinking of your projects, or about what will be happening later in the day. Just stay in the moment and feel the refreshing pleasure of the water moving across your skin, and the dirt and grease of the previous day falling away. You can mindfully get dressed and be glad you have the clothes you need for the day just sitting in your drawer or hanging in a closet nearby. You can walk a few steps to the refrigerator and take out some food for breakfast. Eat your food slowly and mindfully, fully enjoying the flavors and textures of each bite.

Then later, when you take the car, bus, or train to work, you can take joy in how magical it is to just sit down on a little platform while the vehicle does all the work to transport you to your destination. While you travel down the smooth road someone else has built for your convenience, you can marvel at the beauty of nature passing by, the rhythms in the landscape, and the patterns of the passing cars.

When you get out of the car and walk to the entrance of your workplace don't start overplanning or fearing your workday. Instead, stay in the present moment by following your breath and your steps, and be happy you have a job that serves a useful purpose for your community. Then open the door to your workplace, where you can begin anew to treat your fellow workers with kindness, respect, and compassion.

THE ULTIMATE DIMENSION

Buddhism teaches there are two dimensions of reality. The first is called the historical dimension, the conventional way of looking at the universe in terms of form, space, and time. Buddha said that the designations of things and people as coming and going, having a beginning and an end, and separate, independent selves are simply conventional "signs" that we use to describe things in the historical dimension.

The other dimension of reality, in which all things also exist, is called the ultimate dimension. In this dimension, nothing ever truly ceases to exist—everything just transforms into different forms at various times. The earlier section on birth and death (pages 95–99) described the modern scientific principles of the conservation of energy (the first law of thermodynamics) and the transformative properties of matter, time, space, and energy ($E = MC^2$). Twenty-five hundred years ago, Buddha had already recognized that there is an ultimate dimension in which matter (form), time, space, and energy are not absolutes; that all these elements are in a constant state of transformation, which he called "signlessness." When we understand this ultimate dimension, we no longer have to fear impermanence. We feel a sense of joy, peace, and liberation, because we understand that everything, including us and our loved ones, exist in an ultimate state of transformation and will always be here. Buddha called this insight "no death, no fear," a state of enlightenment that is also called Nirvana.

CHAPTER SIX

Mindful Art

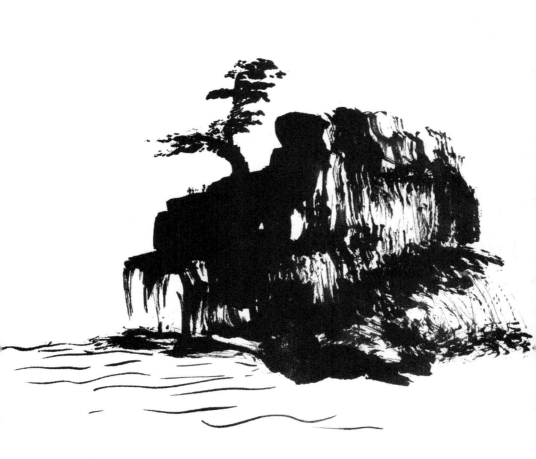

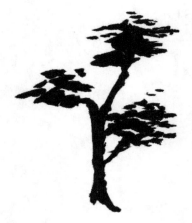

This chapter contains a variety of examples of what I call "mindful art," which is art that stimulates both the artist and the consumers of art to stay mindfully engaged in the present moment while either making or appreciating the artwork. The majority of examples used in this chapter emphasize works by artists in the Zen tradition. Although the art forms of dance and music are discussed, most of the examples cited include artworks that can be reproduced in print. These include samples of calligraphy, painting, sculpture, photography, literature, poetry, song lyrics, Zen rock gardens, stained glass art, and ceramics.

Experiencing great art usually puts a person in a positive state of mind, often associated with emotions like happiness, tranquility, or a sense of wonder. Like other forms of meditation, art appreciation and art making are here-and-now experiences that can help heal a person's mind, body, and spirit. So they are superb mindful activities.

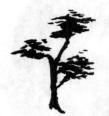

PARTICIPATING IN THE ARTS

Participation in art is a type of mindfulness that is both natural and healthy. Ellen Dissanayake's book *Art and Intimacy: How the Arts Began* (University of Washington Press, 2000) presents anthropological evidence that we are conditioned from an early age to participate in art, and that the arts serve a vital role in helping to bind communities of people together, thereby conferring a healthy survival advantage.

Drawing is a type of art that most people have had some experience doing, having at least tried it when they were young. In *The Zen of Seeing* (Vintage, 1973), artist and writer Frederick Franck writes very poetically about how the act of drawing can be a type of meditation:

What really happens when seeing and drawing become *seeing/*

drawing is that awareness and attention become constant and undivided, become contemplation. *Seeing/drawing* is not a self-indulgence, a "pleasant hobby," but a discipline of awareness, of unwavering attention to a world which is fully alive . . . It is a discipline of *pointed mindfulness* as such, persevered *in* to the point where the *in*-sight breaks through . . . Eye, heart, hand become one with what is seen and drawn, things are seen as they are—in their "isness."

If you are artistically inclined, pick up a drawing pencil or a paintbrush and give *seeing/drawing* a try. It's fun and relaxing, and may also produce interesting insights. There are many other examples of mindful art presented in this chapter. So, don't be shy about trying your hand at more than one art form. As the popular saying goes, "Be smart, make art."

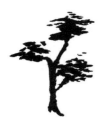

CREATIVITY, CURIOSITY, AND SPONTANEITY

Creativity is a necessary ingredient for producing art. Polymath Jacob Bronowski's creative research and writings spanned the spectrum of the arts and sciences, including mathematics, physics, biology, anthropology, visual art, literature, and poetry. Bronowski defined creativity as the process of organizing things or thoughts into new relationships. In *A Sense of the Future* (MIT Press, 1978), he wrote that a person becomes creative when he finds "a likeness between things which were thought not alike before, and this gives him a sense at the same time of richness and of understanding. The creative mind is a mind that looks for unexpected likenesses." When meditating, the mind is very still and old patterns of thought are suppressed, so new relationships and unexpected likenesses become more apparent. This is why creative ideas occur more frequently during and right after meditation. Therefore, the capacity to make or appreciate art is enhanced by the practice of meditation, whether the art form is music, painting, poetry, literature, or dance.

Artists (and scientists) have an innate inquisitiveness about the mysteries of life. The German novelist Hermann Hesse wrote about this in *Narcissus and Goldmund* (1930). Referring to Goldmund, the sculpture artist in the novel, Hesse writes, "One thing, however did become clear to him—why so many perfect works of art did not please him at all . . . They lacked the most essential thing—mystery. That was what dreams and truly great works of art had in common: mystery." Albert Einstein, who was an accomplished violin player as well as a physicist, wrote, "The most beautiful emotion we can experience is the mysterious. It is the fundamental emotion that stands at the cradle of all true art and science."

For both artists and scientists, creativity and curiosity goes hand-in-hand with spontaneity—where curiosity about new ideas is spontaneously acted upon to create novel associations. Zen writers talk about the value of approaching activities with a childlike "beginner's mind" that sees things as new and wondrous, not just assumes the old associations. As Pablo Picasso famously said, "Every child is an artist. The problem is how to remain an artist once we grow up." Albert Einstein wrote, "There are two ways to live your life. One is as though nothing is a miracle. The other is as though everything is a miracle." People with this type of mind enjoy exploring the world. They may spontaneously recognize a chance unexpected event and give it new emphasis, which may then give rise to a unique work of art or science.

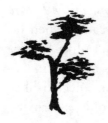

NATURAL, HARMONIOUS, ELEMENTAL ART

Zen art often takes as its subject simple, harmonious, elemental objects found in nature, to help us see the miraculous in the mundane. Alan Watts, in *The Way of Zen* (Vintage Books, 1957), writes, "the expression of Zen in the arts gives us one of the most direct ways of understanding it . . . The favorite subjects of Zen artists, whether painters or poets, are what we should call natural, concrete, and secular things." A perfect example is the art of the Japanese rock garden. See Figure 3 on the following page.

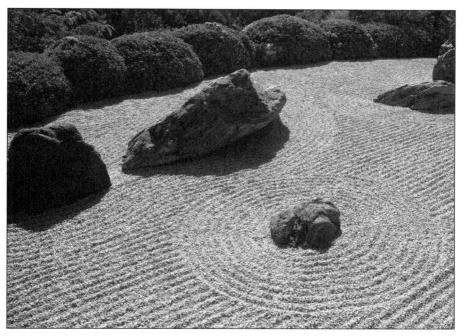

FIGURE 3. Zen Rock Garden at Japanese Friendship Garden,
Balboa Park, San Diego, California.

The garden's rugged simplicity and clarity evokes a sense of peaceful timelessness.

Photography is one of the art forms that can capture the natural essence of our world. The harmony and beauty of nature is the subject of the photograph (Plate 2) on page 182, which shows two different species of birds, a crane and a seagull, both perched harmoniously together on a tree branch in the middle of a lake.

The photograph (Plate 3) on page 183 portrays a lovely yellow lotus blossom. In the Buddhist tradition, the lotus flower has special symbolic meaning. The lotus flower grows out of the mud from the bottom of a pond; as it grows upward toward the light, its colorful petals unfold. This symbolically represents the capacity of people to transform the mud of human suffering into the beauty of spiritual enlightenment.

More beautiful Zen photographs of simple, elemental subjects can be seen in Alan Watts's book *Zen: The Supreme Experience* (Vega, 2002).

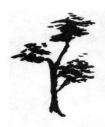

PAINTING, SCULPTURE, AND STAINED GLASS ART

Paintings, statues, and stained glass windows are three wonderful art forms that shine a light into the soul of the artist, and can illuminate the concepts and practices of meditation and Zen.

PAINTING

Chinese and Japanese black ink paintings and calligraphy are other classic examples of Zen art. These paintings celebrate profound qualities of life within a simple form. In *The Way of Zen,* Alan Watts explains that "the characteristic brush line is jagged, gnarled, and irregularly twisting, dashing, or sweeping—always spontaneous rather than predictable . . . The aimless life is the constant theme of Zen art of every kind, expressing the artist's own inner state of going nowhere in a timeless moment."

Furthermore, the manner in which the painting is produced, and the effect that has on the artist who produces it, is as important as the final result. The Zen artist aims to create the painted figure or character in a continuous single stroke, as if the brush were dancing on the page. So, the act of painting becomes a metaphor for a life lived spontaneously in the present moment.

A fine example of Zen calligraphy, *I Have Arrived,* painted by Thich Nhat Hanh, is shown in Plate 4 on page 184. Rosemary KimBal's painting of the Sanskrit symbol for "OM," shown in Figure 4 on the following page, is an excellent example of Zen black ink painting.

Throughout history, many non-Buddhist painters have produced artworks with themes that are consonant with the Zen perspective. A famous example is Rembrandt's Renaissance-era painting entitled *Philosopher in Meditation,* which resides in the Louvre Museum in Paris. This masterpiece depicts an old bearded philosopher sitting in his study with his eyes closed deep in meditation; it is a beautiful representation of the peace and serenity that occurs during meditation. Another Renaissance masterwork is Michelangelo's elaborate Sistine Chapel ceiling painting, *The Creation of Adam.* This iconic painting shows Adam reaching toward

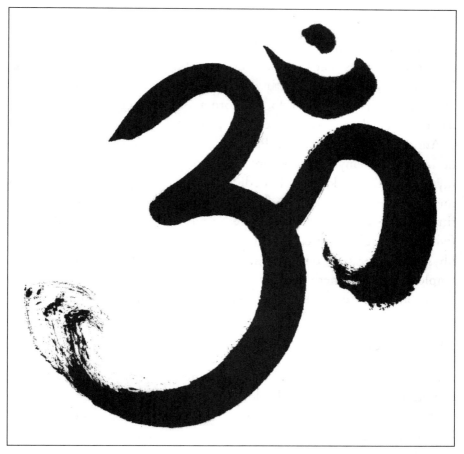

FIGURE 4. *Om* by Rosemary KimBal.

Sanskrit symbol for OM, the original vibration of creation.

God, with Adam's index finger nearly touching the index finger of God's outstretched arm. To me, this is a metaphor for the Zen concept of mankind's capacity to understand and touch the ultimate dimension.

Contemporary Zen artist Rosemary KimBal's painting entitled *Courage* is a stunning work of art mounted high on the wall in the lobby of Scripps Memorial Hospital in Encinitas, California. See Plate 5 on page 185 for photographs of this colorful painting. It was produced to be a form of "healing art" that gives courage to patients who enter the hospital to battle serious illnesses.

SCULPTURE

Sculpture art is well represented in the Zen tradition by the multitude of Buddha statues that have been created. They usually depict a smiling Buddha in the act of meditating. One of my favorites is located at Deer Park Monastery in Escondido, California. A photograph of this magnificent statue (Plate 6) can be seen on page 186.

Another fascinating statue (Plate 7) is pictured on page 187. This statue is one of many classic sculptured representations of Asclepius, the mythological Greek god of medicine whose compassion and skillful means of healing were legendary. In ancient Greek and Roman times, throughout the Mediterranean area, there were scores of health spas (what we would now call wellness centers) dedicated to that famous physician. Therapeutic treatments offered at those Temples of Asclepius employed natural methods consisting of special diets, physical exercises, music, and spiritual practices to heal the mind, body, and spirit.

STAINED GLASS

Another type of modern-day "temple of healing" is the Ocean of Peace Meditation Hall at Deer Park Monastery in Escondido, California. Plate 1 on page 181, referred to earlier in the book, is a photograph of the beautiful stained glass window that adorns that meditation hall. The three Sanskrit words (*smrti, samadhi, prajna*) inscribed in this stained glass work of art remind everyone of the three-part healing practices of mindfulness, concentration, and insight.

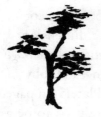

MUSIC

Music is one of mankind's most appreciated and celebrated art forms. Music can touch people's souls and transcend the normal barriers of age, language, and culture. As we saw in Chapter 4, music can also be therapy to soothe the mind, heal the body, and exalt the spirit. Classical music compositions, like Bach's *Brandenburg Concertos* and Vivaldi's *Four Seasons,* are satisfying works of art that have been performed to the delight of audiences for centuries. Many other styles of music can be equally evocative. I have experienced the exhilarating rush and joyful energy that comes from playing concert band music, jazz, blues, and popular music with fellow musicians.

Certain musical instruments like the flute, sitar, and acoustic guitar are particularly capable of producing an intrinsically meditative sound. See Plate 8 on page 187 of talented musician Adrienne Nims playing her Chinese bamboo flute in the midst of a bamboo garden. (Adrienne may be heard playing the Native American wood flute on Track 1 of the *Teaching Meditation* audio CD that accompanies this book.)

The lyrics of some of the songs in the great American songbook mirror several key ideas that are part of the Zen perspective discussed in Chapter 3. For instance, the concept of mindfully enjoying the present moment is the point of a James Taylor song entitled "Secret O' Life," wherein Taylor says, "The secret of life is enjoying the passage of time."

The practice of smiling to transform negative states of mind is reflected in the song "Smile." The song's lyrics, written by John Turner and Geoffrey Parsons, advise that you should "light up your face with gladness . . . although a tear may be ever so near." (The melody of this song was composed by comedian Charlie Chaplin, a man who obviously knew the importance of smiling.) Similar lyrical advice is contained in the lyrics of a famous song from the musical *Bye, Bye Birdie,* which tells us that "gray skies are gonna clear up" if we just "put on a happy face."

Zen-like advice that the quality of your life path matters more than achieving some future goal carries the same sentiment that is embodied in the title of a song written by jazz musicians Trummy Young and Sy Oliver that advises, "T'Ain't What You Do (It's the Way That You Do It)."

Louis Armstrong sang expressively about seeing "trees of green" and "red roses, too" in a famous recording of "What a Wonderful World." This is a great song about being in touch with the wonders of nature.

Meditation and centering the mind appears to be the point of Horace Silver's song "Permit Me to Introduce You to Yourself," which has the following lyrics: "There's a meeting place where you can get together. And you'll find it in the center of your mind."

The song "Happiness Is Here and Now" is frequently sung by the monks, nuns, and lay people at Deer Park and Plum Village in France. This song can be heard on a music CD produced at Plum Village called *A Basket of Plums*. The lyrics, printed below, of this simple but deep song explain that happiness is enhanced by slowing down and focusing your awareness on what is happening in the here and now.

Happiness Is Here and Now
THICH NHAT HANH AND PLUM VILLAGE

Happiness is here and now.
    I have dropped my worry.
Nowhere to go; nothing to do;
    no longer in a hurry.
Happiness is here and now.
    I have dropped my worry.
Somewhere to go; something to do;
    but I don't need to hurry.

"Happiness Is Here and Now," from *A Basket of Plums: Songs for the Practice of Mindfulness*, Josef Emet, ed., reprinted with permission of Parallax Press, Berkeley, CA; www.parallax.org.

I have composed songs for six jazz CDs; the two most recent discs are *Mindful* (2003) and *Watering the Seeds* (2005). The lyrics of two of the songs from those CDs appear on the following pages. The first song, "Every Day Above Ground," contains insights about coping with the impermanence of life.

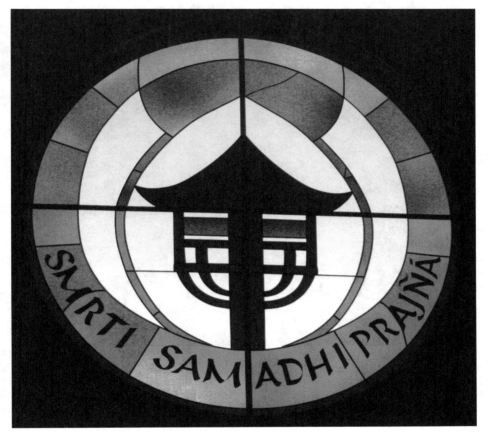

Plate 1. Stained glass window in the Ocean of Peace Meditation Hall, Deer Park Monastery, Escondido, California.

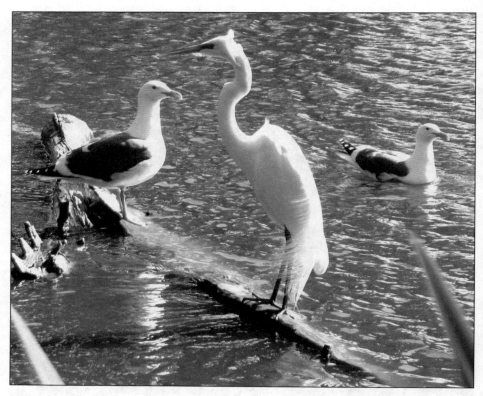

Plate 2. Equanimity in nature.

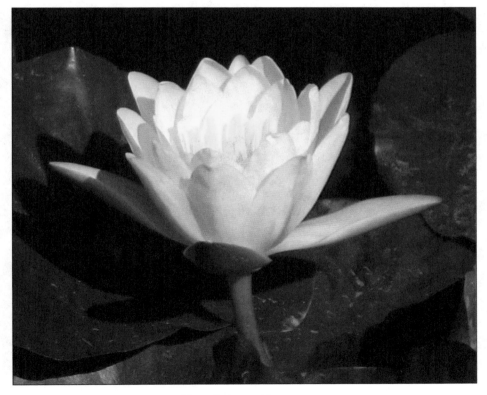

Plate 3. Lotus blossom.

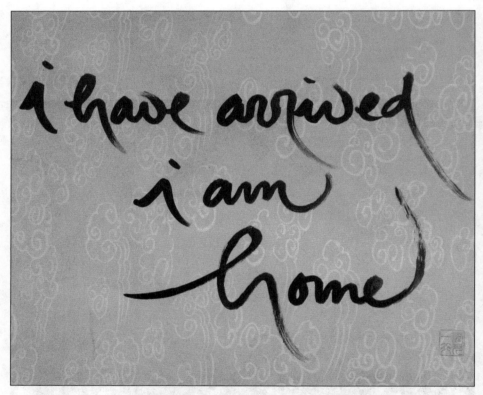

Plate 4. *I Have Arrived* by Thich Nhat Hanh.

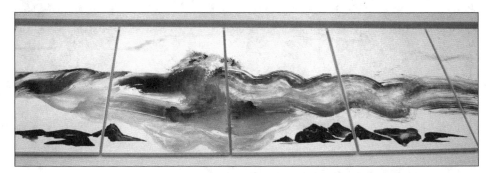

Plate 5. *Courage* by Rosemary KimBal.

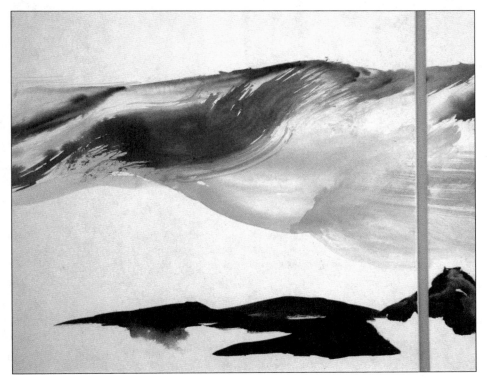

Close-up portion of the painting.

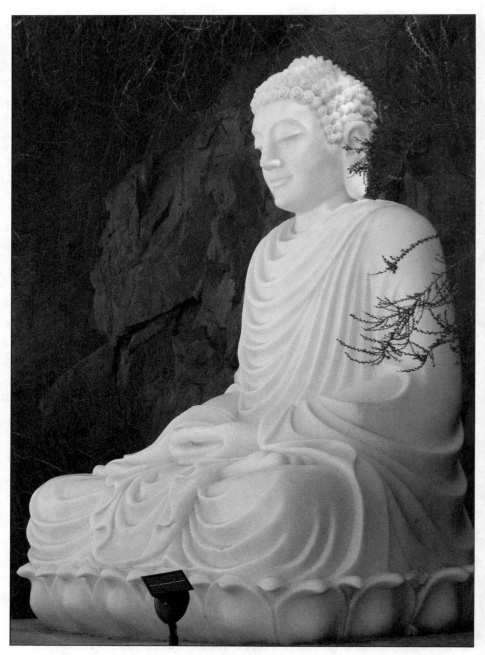

Plate 6. Buddha statue at Deer Park Monastery.

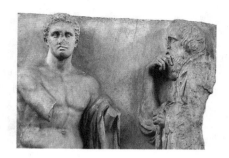

Plate 7. Ailing young man being helped by Asclepius, the ancient Greek god of medicine, Athens, Greece.

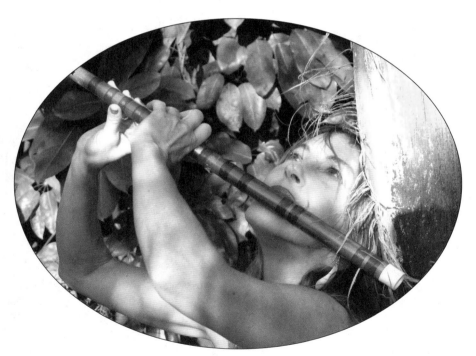

Plate 8. Bamboo flute being played by Adrienne Nims.

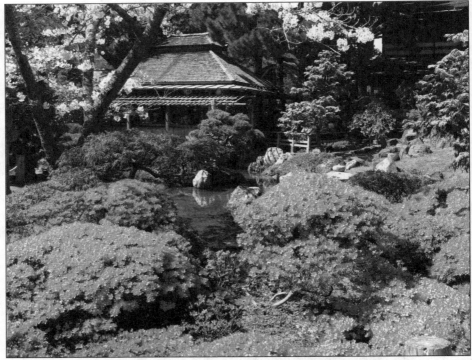

Plate 9. Tea house at the Japanese Tea Garden in Golden Gate Park, San Francisco.

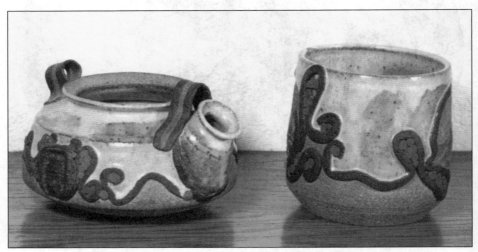

Plate 10. Teapot and bowl with colored clay by Lana Wilson.

Every Day Above Ground
BY GABRIEL WEISS

My hair's gotten grayer and my belly just seems to grow . . .
    and I'm slow.
My troubles are spread out on a world wide web of woe . . .
    feeling low.
'Cause nothing lasts forever and what's good in life
    eventually will go.

My brother's got cancer and the chemo is tough.
Fellow workers are greedy, and they're treating me rough.
Believe me. I never thought that life was fair.
But don't despair.
'Cause I heard some wisdom spoken
by a man whose life was wrecked beyond repair.
This was his prayer . . .

Every day above ground is a very good day.
Every day above ground gives me reasons to say,
"Every day above ground, wipe the tears away.
'Cause every day above ground is a good day, baby."
Don't think about the past, or the future forecast.
Start living in the here and now.

You should know that now's the time.
But, it's easy to forget.
And then you're thinking 'bout the past or the future forecast.
Start living in the here and now!

My hearing is going and my eyes are not keen.
My knees are arthritic, and this backache is mean.
Oh, and baby, I never told you we would be rich.
Ain't life a bitch?

But, consider the alternative, and I don't think I'd really
    choose to switch.
This is my niche. So . . .

Every day above ground is a very good day.
Every day above ground gives me reasons to say,
"Every day above ground, wipe the tears away.
'Cause every day above ground is a good day, baby."
Don't think about the past, or the future forecast.
Start living in the here and now.
That's how . . .
you can see you got a great life
when you're living here and now.
Right now!

The lyrics of the next song, "Bluesology," illustrate how music (in this case, blues music) can be used as music therapy to reduce pain, fear, and stress.

Bluesology
BY GABRIEL WEISS

Skiing down the snowdrifts, riding back up on the chairlifts,
    past the snowplows;
the weather it was storming and the icicles were forming on
    my eyebrows
    and my lips.
My fingers and toes were nearly all froze.
I felt like a suffering sack of woes.

Sierra winds were screaming and powdered snow was
    streaming in a flurry.
Trapped within a blizzard, my breath quivered as I shivered,
    full of worry
    and of pain.

Then it came to me, this Bluesology.
It melted my soul and set me free.

Here's how to take shelter from the blizzard of thoughts that
    swirl through your mind.
Take all of your anger, fears, and thoughts that are unkind,
and sing them as Blues, and your stress will unwind.

If Blues are what you're feeling, take advantage of the healing
    in the music.
Your spirit can be warming while the outside world is
    storming if you use it.
    And it's free.
Fear transformed through me
    to Bluesology.
And that was my music therapy.

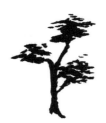

DANCING MOLECULES AND THE TEA CEREMONY

Dancing can serve the useful purpose of being a kind of mating ritual. However, dancing can also be a wonderful form of movement meditation. When two people are dancing together, they are not doing it in order to finally arrive at a particular place on the dance floor, as they would on a journey. When people are dancing, the journey itself is the point. So with dance, just as in any form of meditation, the point of life is always arrived at in the immediate moment.

Performance dance art celebrates the beauty of human movement, as well as the joy of being in the moment. Dances created by master choreographers like Martha Graham, José Limón, George Balanchine, Alvin Ailey, and Jerome Robbins are exhilarating to watch. Seeing dances like these helps to inspire us to discover the immense possibilities of rhythmical movement and the physical capabilities of the human body.

DANCING MOLECULES

Dances can be fashioned around themes that are concrete, fanciful, or abstract. While at Stanford Medical School, I wrote and directed a dance movie entitled *Protein Synthesis: An Epic on the Cellular Level* (1971), in which many people danced out the process of molecules interacting to form proteins inside of a cell. Figure 5 below is a photograph that was taken while filming the movie. The aim of making this movie was to better teach the current scientific model of protein synthesis in a way that went beyond the static drawings in scientific texts, and to have fun doing it. The dynamic molecular reactions were portrayed as a beautiful dance of molecules. It showed both the interconnectedness and randomness of the process, and how nature in us is all in all.

As described by Ellen Dissanayake in *Art and Intimacy: How the Arts Began,* the original purpose of dance was to help bind a community of people together and help them feel how they were interconnected. Dance has functioned this way in tribal rituals from the beginning of human civilization. It is clear to me that the *Protein Synthesis* dance event we put together had the amazing effect of binding together the community of Stanford students who participated in the dance. In fact, thirty-five years after the original event, I went back to Stanford and met with

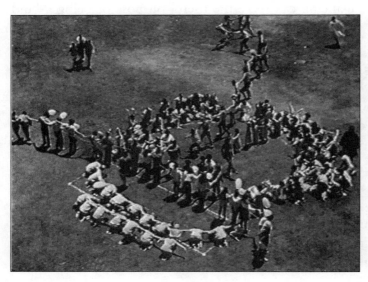

FIGURE 5.
Protein Synthesis: An Epic on the Cellular Level, Stanford University, 1971.

People dancing out the process of molecules interacting to form proteins inside of a cell.

former teachers and students there who were still talking about it. Indeed, *Protein Synthesis: An Epic on the Cellular Level* is currently enjoying a new life on the Internet. If you go to the website YouTube.com, you can see the original film, and also look at several other film projects that were inspired by our movie to create dances in the same genre.

THE TEA CEREMONY

A completely different type of ritual that binds people together in Japan is the tea ceremony, which has evolved into a form of high art. Alan Watts, in *Zen: The Supreme Experience,* writes, "The tea ceremony in particular has been central to Zen because it is like opera in the sense that opera involves many arts—music, drama, staging, ballet, and so on. The people who developed the tea ceremony became masters of aesthetics, because every single one of the arts—ceramics, bronze-making, painting, architecture, gardening, the cultivation of rocks—collects around the ceremonial."

The tea ceremony traditionally takes place in a separate tea house that is situated in a beautifully landscaped garden. An impressive Japanese tea garden located in San Francisco's Golden Gate Park (see Plate 9 on page 188). Plate 10 on page 188 is a photograph of a contemporary Zen-like teapot and bowl created by ceramic artist Lana Wilson.

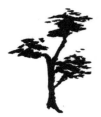

LITERATURE AND POETRY

The language arts of literature and poetry are powerful ways to express the principles of Zen and the meaning of meditation.

LITERATURE

In American literature, Jack Kerouac, who became a Buddhist, was a popular Beat Generation author. His 1958 novel *The Dharma Bums* (Penguin Classics, 2006 edition) introduced many Americans to the concepts of Zen. The novel is based loosely on Kerouac's association with

Zen poet Gary Snyder, who is represented by the book's character Japhy. In *The Dharma Bums,* Japhy would often quote Buddha: "All life is suffering." Of Japhy, Kerouac writes, "He learned Chinese and Japanese and became an Oriental scholar and discovered the greatest Dharma Bums of them all, the Zen lunatics of China and Japan." Ray, the protagonist in the story, tries to achieve enlightenment through the study of Buddhist philosophy. He and Japhy share some wild adventures in the great outdoors, hiking and mountain climbing.

One of my favorite novelists is Kurt Vonnegut. In his last book, *A Man Without a Country* (Seven Stories Press, 2005), Vonnegut expresses a Zen-like joy of living in the present moment this way: "We are dancing animals. How beautiful it is to get up and go out and do something. We are here on earth to fart around."

John Steinbeck was awarded the Nobel Prize in Literature. He is another gritty American author who, like the Zen philosophers, could describe a mundane scene in such a way as to raise our awareness of how sublimely beautiful ordinary life is. A good example is the opening line from his novel *Cannery Row* (Penguin Classics, [1945] 1994): "Cannery Row in Monterey in California is a poem, a stink, a grating noise, a quality of light, a tone, a habit, a nostalgia, a dream."

Hermann Hesse, who wrote *Siddhartha* (1922) and *Journey to the East* (1932), was a German novelist who was quite aware of Eastern spiritual ideas—such as Buddha's teaching about the five constantly changing aggregates of the self. Hesse's novel *Steppenwolf* (Picador, 2002), written in 1927, contains the metaphor of game pieces on a chessboard, which represent the changing nature of the self composed of a multiplicity of pieces. In the following excerpt from *Steppenwolf,* the novel's main character, Harry Haller, has just entered the Magic Theatre, a surreal place where behind each door Harry encounters a different fantastical episode that forces him to confront the contradictions of his so-called personality. In one of the rooms, Harry finds a man sitting on the floor in Eastern fashion in front of a chessboard filled with a variety of curious game pieces. He looks up at Harry and says, "The mistaken and unhappy notion that man is an enduring unity is known to you. It is also known that man consists of a multitude of souls, of numerous selves . . . We demonstrate to anyone whose soul has fallen to pieces that he can rearrange these pieces of a previous self in what order he pleases, and so attain an endless multiplicity of moves in the game of life."

POETRY

The art of poetry is very much aligned with the sensibilities of Zen in that poets attempt to simplify language down to the bare essentials needed to express the ideas and feelings they are trying to communicate. This simplification of language is highly evolved in the poetic form of the Japanese haiku. A haiku is a poem composed of just three lines. A haiku, like most Zen art, attempts to express universal themes through simple natural images.

Matsuo Basho (1643–1694) is considered by many to be one of the finest writers of Japanese haiku. In *Zen Buddhism: Selected Writings of D. T. Suzuki,* Daisetz Suzuki describes Basho as "a great travelling poet, a most passionate lover of nature—a kind of nature troubadour." One of Basho's best-known poems, "Old Pond," is printed below.

Old Pond
BY MATSUO BASHO

Old pond
A frog leaps
The sound of water

"The Five Insights" is a poem I wrote. While not a haiku, it attempts to describe in as simple a form as possible the core Zen principles of impermanence, interconnectedness, nonattachment, compassion, and mindfulness. The following poem was designed to be easily memorized so it could be used as a gatha for walking meditation.

The Five Insights
BY GABRIEL WEISS

I., I., N., C.
I eye 'n' see
the nature of reality.

I., I., N., C.
and mindfully
looking deeply I am free.

"Watering the Seeds" is another (somewhat wordier) poem I wrote for use during walking meditation. I later composed a gospel-like melody for it and turned the poem into a song that became the title of one of my music CDs. A recital of "Watering the Seeds" can be heard on Track 3 of the *Teaching Meditation* audio CD that accompanies this book.

Watering the Seeds
BY GABRIEL WEISS

Watering the good seeds in the garden of my mind,
digging up the roots of suffering, this is what I find.
Try letting go of grudges, hatred, jealousy, and fear.
All things are impermanent. So, while we are here,
we're dwelling in the wonders of the here and now.

Here's how.
Be joy, compassion, forgiveness, and peace.
Awareness in the present, we avow . . .
to be joy, compassion, kindness, and peace.
We're inter-being in the here and now.

Mindful and completely here,
we're concentrating and the wisdom's clear.
We're all connected in the here and now.

CHAPTER SEVEN

The Nature of Reality and Consciousness

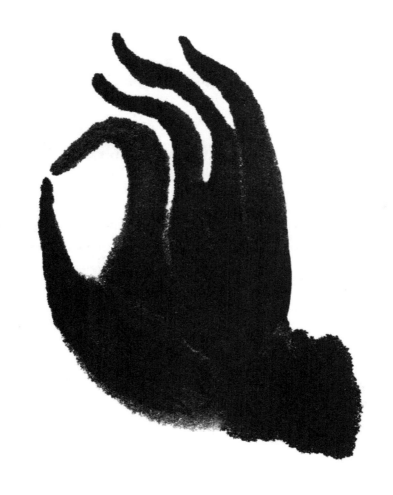

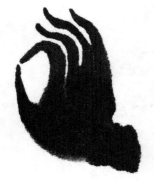

Meditation is both a healing art and a science of mind and body. This final chapter explains key aspects of Western science's views on the nature of reality and how the mind works, and compares and contrasts these with Eastern insights about meditation and Zen. You will see how the scientific view of reality and the Zen perspective outlined earlier in this book are not inconsistent but, in fact, inform and complement one another. This neuroscientific description of how the mind works includes: the surprising role that feelings play in life regulation; how it is that we have the capacity for consciousness awareness; and the mechanisms by which we are able to learn and acquire wisdom. Lastly, this chapter reveals the neurobiology of how meditation affects the mind and enhances our health and well-being.

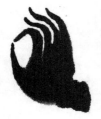

SCIENCE AND ZEN

British mathematician, scientist, and humanitarian Jacob Bronowski, who was mentioned previously in the book, worked in the 1960s at the Salk Institute for Biological Studies in La Jolla, California. There, he wrote the BBC television documentary series and book called *The Ascent of Man,* wherein he insisted all science is philosophy. He called it "natural philosophy." He wrote, "My ambition here has been to create a philosophy that is all of one piece . . . For me the understanding of nature has as its goal the understanding of human nature, and of the human condition within nature."

It is appealing (and challenging) to try to put together a natural philosophy of life that is consistent with available observations and experimental results. The way the natural elements fit together can, as Albert Einstein described it, "take the form of rapturous amazement at the harmony of natural law . . . a sort of intoxicated joy and amazement at the beauty and grandeur of this world . . . This joy is the feeling from which true scientific research draws its spiritual sustenance."

WE WILL NEVER UNDERSTAND IT ALL

However, all models of reality, no matter how grand and beautiful, must be understood to be imperfect reflections of the true reality. We will never understand it all. In fact, we still have an incomplete understanding of some of the most basic elements of nature. For example, neither science nor any other field of study has yet provided a compelling explanation for what empowers energy and gives it the capacity to transform matter. One of the greatest physics teachers of the twentieth century, Richard Feynman, PhD, wrote, "It is important to realize that in physics today we have no knowledge of what energy is."

Siddhartha Gautama also taught that any view of reality is imperfect. He said, "What you see and hear comprises only a small part of reality. If you take it to be the whole of reality, you will end up having a distorted picture. A person on the path must keep a humble, open heart, acknowledging that his understanding is incomplete . . . Humility and open-mindedness are two conditions necessary for making progress on the path."

NEXUS OF SCIENCE AND ZEN

The perspectives of both science and Zen Buddhism can help us to look more deeply into the nature of reality. Zen takes a scientific-like view of causation. Zen teaches that all objects and thoughts are "formations." Formations only become manifest when sufficient preceding conditions are present. This is so, because that is so. This principle also goes by several interchangeable Buddhist names: interconnectedness, interdependency, dependent co-arising, and emptiness. Most scientists take a similar deterministic view of how the universe works.

Science and Buddhism share similar methods of investigating reality and forming conclusions. The Dalai Lama has written, "The Buddhist approach to knowledge is similar to that of modern science. Results should be determined through analysis, examining the evidence with reason."

In his introduction to *Buddhism and Science* (Columbia University Press, 2003), Buddhist scholar and practitioner B. Alan Wallace, PhD, explains that Buddhism is like science in that it endeavors to be a "body of systematic knowledge about the natural world" that can be tested by experience. In the same book, there is an essay by theoretical physicist David Finkelstein comparing the Buddhist concept of emptiness to the scientific theory of relativity, and an essay by physicist William Ames, comparing the Buddhist concept of emptiness to modern scientific quantum theory.

DIFFERENCES BETWEEN SCIENCE AND ZEN

There are, however, some noteworthy differences between science and Zen. Science regards individual experience as too anecdotal to be considered noteworthy of analysis. Whereas, as you may remember, Zen Buddhism proposes that individual experience should be the "laboratory" wherein one makes a judgment for oneself as to the validity of Buddhist theories. The importance of reconciling both the objective and subjective understanding of the world is expressed by this quote from *A Path with Heart* by Jack Kornfield: "The greatest lesson I have learned is that the universal must be wedded to the personal to be fulfilled in our spiritual life."

Another distinction is that, whereas Zen has an overarching perspective that could be called a worldview, science's description of reality is too incomplete to call it a worldview. In "Life as a Laboratory," one of the essays in *Buddhism and Science,* astrophysicist Piet Hut writes, "For an approach to reality to be comprehensive enough to call it a worldview, at the very least such a view should have room for human life, meaning, dignity, responsibility, and other aspects of what it means to be human . . . But the current scientific description of reality leaves out far too much to deserve the name worldview."

INTERCONNECTEDNESS, IMPERMANENCE, ENTROPY, AND EVOLUTION

Despite these differences, science and Zen have a lot in common. Like science, the practice of Zen is meant to be validated by the empiric evidence of the experienced world. In "Life as a Laboratory" Dr. Hut writes,

"I relished the Buddhist emphasis on its view of reality as something utterly concrete and accessible, something that could be experienced here and now, by anybody—not something to be stumbled upon only in the afterlife, if one lived a good enough life in blind faith."

The principles of Zen are generally consistent with, and do not contradict, the experimental observations and associated theories of science. For instance, the Zen principle of interconnectedness is consistent with scientific observations that have repeatedly demonstrated that the forces of nature and the physical objects in the universe interact in interdependent ways.

Scientific theories are also consistent with the Zen insight of impermanence. The imperative of impermanence is partly explained by the scientific principle of entropy (the second law of thermodynamics), which describes the tendency for natural systems to become more disorganized and dissipated over time.

Counterbalancing entropy, but also contributing to the process of change in an impermanent universe, is the phenomenon of evolution. Evolution requires energy and, over time, creates change in the direction of more organization of matter and energy. Evolution occurs through a process that biologist Charles Darwin described as natural selection based on survival advantage in a given environment. While plant and animal evolution occurs one small genetic change at a time, the diversity it produces is enormous. The phenomenon of evolution occurs on many different levels. One level is classical Darwinian evolution of plant and animal species over eons of time. There are also other types of evolution, including the cultural evolution of human civilization; the evolution of our brains over our lifetime; the evolution of the ever-changing planet earth; and the evolution of matter as the various atomic elements are assembled over billions of years within the intense nuclear reactions in stars.

CHANCE "MISTAKES"

The importance of what seems like chance events, or what some might call mistakes, cannot be overlooked. While there is some disagreement on this point, which we will discuss, life is not just mechanistic systems that play out over time in a predetermined way. Indeed, the very essence of evolution and development of new species seems to require random mistakes in the copying of DNA and mistakes in the manufacture of proteins to occur. Occasionally, these random, quantum mistakes produce new and better adaptations to an ever-changing surrounding environment. This is the biological equivalent of the Heisenberg uncertainty principle, one of the central principles of modern physics. This uncertainty principle should inform us not to be so afraid of making mistakes. To err is human and completely natural. We can recover from mistakes and often be better off afterward than we were before.

OTHER SCIENTIFIC PRINCIPLES

Other key scientific principles consistent with Zen include the first law of thermodynamics, which is also called the conservation of energy, quantum mechanics, and Einstein's famous equation relating energy and matter as $E = MC^2$. Aspects of these other scientific principles were mentioned earlier in Chapter 3 in the section "Birth and Death."

REALISM AND UNCERTAINTY

What did Einstein, Spinoza, and Buddha have in common? They shared an awe-inspiring reverence for the laws of nature that govern the way the universe works. They also shared an optimism that it is possible for humans to discover those laws and benefit from applying that knowledge. While they thought that the laws of nature were possibly a reflection of a divine order, Einstein, Spinoza, and Buddha all rejected the idea of a God who takes an interest and intervenes in the affairs of individual humans.

Einstein, Spinoza, and Buddha would be called realists, in the sense that they believed that there is an objective reality that can become apparent to us if we look deeply enough. These three wise men also believed in a deterministic universe, which works on the basis of a balance of forces determining the outcome of an event. This is so, because that is so. (Or this is not so, because that is not so. Or this is so, because that is not so, and visa versa.)

This is in contradistinction to the approach taken by the next generation of physicists who came to prominence after Einstein's theory of relativity had been accepted by the scientific community. Scientists like Werner Heisenberg and Erwin Schrödinger proposed that the latest scientific experiments looking into the nature of subatomic particles, light, and electromagnetism led to the conclusion that, at the most basic level, there is a randomness of action such that a particular object or event can never be said to exist with certainty, but only within a mathematical range of probability. Einstein often said he could not accept this view because it would imply that God was playing dice. Einstein's opponents say that part of the reason we can never discern objects or events with certainty is because the act of observing an event changes the event. This is particularly true when we try to observe things like subatomic particles and photons of light. These physicists believe that the knowledge we have of the universe is based solely on observations that are inherently uncertain. This is quite apart from any notion of seeking to understand a true objective reality.

Like his hero, Sir Isaac Newton, Einstein believed in the concept of an objective reality that science attempts to understand. But, unlike Newton and all of the scientists that came after Newton, Einstein realized that the entities of time and space are not absolute and unchangeable. Einstein's great creative insight was that the measurements of time and space change relative to the motion of an object. Time and space are linked together in what Einstein called "the fabric of space-time." Space and time measurements of an object are always related to the object's motion relative to a given frame of reference. Einstein's theory of relativity allows one to mathematically calculate this relationship between space and time.

Einstein worked for the last half of his career trying to develop mathematical equations that would provide a complete theory to explain all natural phenomena. He called this "the quest for a unified field theory." Einstein was never successful, but he said he thought that was because there was a force or element of natural law that had yet to be discovered. And that, once found, it would explain what had heretofore appeared to be random outcomes in some physics experiments.

The latest attempt to develop a unified field theory is the mathematics of the string theory, also called M-theory. Theoretical physicist Edward Witten has made major contributions to this field. A number of contemporary physicists who understand the mathematics say this theory does work to mathematically unify the known forces of nature, including quantum mechanics and gravity. However, to date, there has been no experimental evidence to validate this theory. And the ten or eleven dimensions postulated by this theory are difficult to understand and impossible to visualize. So, until there is experimental evidence to back up the theory, many physicists will remain skeptical that the string theory really explains it all.

I find myself attracted to the view of the realists that there is an objective reality that humans can attempt to comprehend. I also stand in awe of the enormous body of knowledge that humans have discovered about how the universe works, and how it appears to follow certain predictable laws. On the other hand, I acknowledge that, at the level of our own human awareness, our daily life will always contain an element of uncertainty.

For example, we will never be able to calculate with certainty what will occur in the next few seconds, as the moments of our lives pass along. Therefore, we will always have to deal with life as a series of surprises and apparent chance events that generate impermanence, which often leads to suffering. This is why we need to continually practice the skillful means that help shield us from that suffering.

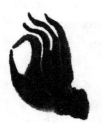

FEELINGS: THE RIPPLE EFFECT

Why do we have feelings? Are feelings simply a byproduct of living, or do they exist for a deeper purpose? Feelings are among the least-well-understood aspects of our inner world. According to Buddhist teachings, feelings are one of the five component elements of a person (the body, perceptions, mental formations, and consciousness being the other four). These elements have overlapping properties. For example, the form of the body strongly influences the function of the other elements. Perceptions, whether correct or incorrect, often generate mental formations.

Buddhist teachings also classify feelings as a type of mental formation. Zen practitioners are usually advised to not dwell on, get caught up in, or take action during the heat of a negative feeling, observing that all feelings simply arise, develop, and pass away.

But, a deeper understanding of feelings and emotions is warranted since they play such a pivotal role in biological regulation. This section will focus on what feelings are, what important purposes they serve, and how they function. Knowing how feelings function can help us become more consciously aware of the presence of positive or negative feelings. The practice of meditation can then transform negative feelings like fear and sorrow, as well as promote positive feelings like joy and wellness.

WHAT ARE FEELINGS FOR?

Antonio Damasio, previously mentioned in Chapter 5, is a neurologist and neuroscientist who has held faculty positions at the University of Southern California, the University of Iowa, and the Salk Institute. In *Looking for Spinoza: Joy, Sorrow, and the Feeling Brain*, Dr. Damasio describes in great depth what feelings are:

> Feelings are the expression of human flourishing or human distress, as they occur in the mind and body. Feelings are not a mere decoration added on to the emotion, something one might keep or discard. Feelings can be and often are revelations of the state of life within the entire organism . . . They translate the ongoing life state in the language of the mind . . . Feelings of pain or pleasure or some quality in between are the bedrock of our minds. We often fail to notice this simple reality because the mental images of the objects and events that surround us, along with the images of the words and sentences that describe them, use up so much of our overburdened attention.

If Damasio is correct, becoming aware of our emotions and feelings can be an important way to assess the general state of our well-being, or lack thereof. After becoming aware of our feelings, we might then be able to transform and let go of negative feelings, or simply dwell in the warm glow of a positive feeling.

TYPES OF FEELINGS

There are different types of feelings and accompanying emotions. There are primary feelings—emotions that may include all gradations of joy and happiness, sadness and sorrow, neutral feelings, anxiety, fear, surprise, contempt, or anger. There are social feelings—emotions like empathy or sympathy, pride, disgust, jealousy, and shame or embarrassment. There are background feelings like energy, fatigue, well-being, malaise, freshness, calm, tension, or anticipation. In *Emotions Revealed* (Holt, 2nd ed., 2007), psychologist Paul Ekman points out that in some situations, we may have a mixture of two or more feelings at the same time, such as surprise and happiness, or sorrow and fear.

HOW DO FEELINGS WORK?

In *Looking for Spinoza,* Damasio writes, "Feelings are perceptions . . . Alongside the perceptions of the body, there is the perception of thoughts with themes consonant with the emotion." Dr. Damasio identifies several relatively small areas in the brain that are responsible for the expression of emotion. These consist of the basal forebrain (a group of structures that lie near the bottom of the front of the brain), parts of the brain stem, and the limbic system (located deep within the brain). Two important structures in the limbic system are the hypothalamus, which is functionally linked to the pituitary gland, and the amygdala, a region of the brain that is especially involved in the processing of stimuli that trigger fear and other emotions. See Figure 6, Anatomy of the Brain, on the following page.

The expression of emotion requires an appropriate external stimulus to be sensed by these areas in the brain. This in turn triggers the firing of nerve synapse pathways (connection points) to the facial muscles and other areas of the body, such as the heart, blood vessels, muscles, adrenal glands, and so on, and the release of certain hormones and peptides that have a chemical effect on the body and a modulating effect on the functioning of neurons in the brain. The combined effect of all of this is to produce in us feelings and the expression of emotion.

PET scans can detect regional differences in brain metabolism. Such

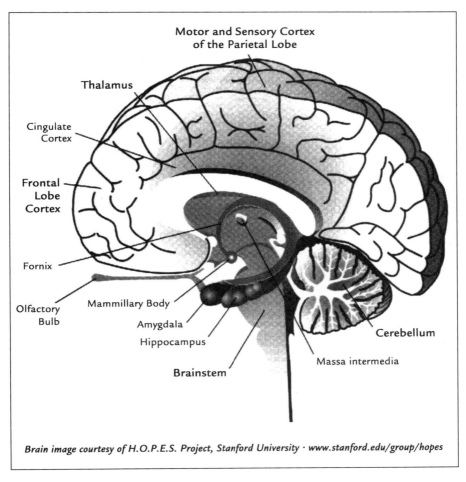

Brain image courtesy of H.O.P.E.S. Project, Stanford University · www.stanford.edu/group/hopes

FIGURE 6. Anatomy of the Brain.

Viewed as if the left half of the brain was cut away to reveal
several internal brain structures.

brain scans have shown that when an emotional state is activated, there
is a distinctive pattern of responses in the brain regions just noted that
are responsible for the various kinds of emotions. There are different patterns seen for happiness versus sadness, versus fear or anger, and so on.

The sequence of events is that there first occurs what Damasio calls
an "emotionally competent stimulus" that induces in us an emotional

state by activating the brain centers and body pathways just described. Sensing those changes then causes us to have internal feelings. Later, due to interaction with our consciousness, we may become consciously aware of those feelings. Becoming conscious of the feelings theoretically might involve what is described as "mapping" an image of that set of neuro-chemical muscular changes in our brain. However, the mechanism of that neurological imaging or mapping has yet to be worked out.

EMOTIONS VERSUS FEELINGS

In one of Damasio's earlier books, *The Feeling of What Happens* (Harcourt, 1999), he writes, "I have proposed that the term 'feeling' should be reserved for the private, mental experience of an emotion, while the term 'emotion' should be used to designate the collection of responses, many of which are publicly observable." And in *Looking for Spinoza*, he elaborates further, "Emotions are actions or movements, many of them public, visible to others as they occur in the face, in the voice, in specific behaviors . . . Feelings, on the other hand, are always hidden, like all mental images always are, unseen to anyone other than their rightful owner, the most private property of the organism in whose brain they occur. Emotions play out in the theater of the body. Feelings play out in the theater of the mind."

In the brain, at the cellular and molecular levels, there are a vast number of activated neural pathways and electrochemical reactions going on at the same time, with many subsystems and neural networks involved. It is too complicated for our awareness to keep track of it all in real time. Feelings, however, can give us an overall sense of how it's all going and if corrective action needs to be taken. Emotions, on the other hand, prepare our bodies for imminent action, and help us to quickly telegraph in a global way our state of being or reaction to other humans. This facilitates important social interaction and group action, and improves our ability to survive.

Studies have shown that emotions come first and feelings then follow. In *Looking for Spinoza*, Damasio references experimental work done by psychologist Paul Ekman: "He asked subjects to move certain muscles of the face in a certain sequence, such that, unbeknownst to the subjects, the expression became one of happiness, or sadness, or fear. The subjects did not know which emotion was being portrayed on their faces. And yet the subjects came to feel the feeling appropriate to the emotion displayed."

So, emotional expression causes us to have internal feelings. Thich Nhat Hanh understands this relationship when he recommends that meditating with a slight smile on your face increases your feeling of happiness. He calls it "mouth yoga." The feeling of happiness occurs as a direct neurological response to moving the muscles of your face into a smiling position.

EMOTIONS: OUR SURVIVAL KIT

Included in the realm of emotional responses are many automatic physiological phenomena that prepare the body to take action, such as to fight, or take flight, or to freeze in response to a perceived threat. In *The Feeling of What Happens,* Damasio explains,

> Emotional responses are the result of a long history of evolutionary fine-tuning. Emotions are part of the bioregulatory devices with which we come equipped to survive. That is why Darwin was able to catalog the emotional expressions of so many species and find consistency in these expressions, and that is why, in different parts of the world and across different cultures, emotions are so easily recognized . . . At their most basic, emotions are part of homeostatic regulation and are poised to avoid the loss of integrity that is a harbinger of death or death itself, as well as to endorse a source of energy, shelter, or sex.

Because emotional expression is so consistent from species to species, it is easy to know when your pet dog is happy, sad, angry, or worried. This also explains why emotions can communicate so much to us about a person from another culture whose spoken language may be unfamiliar. This observation is found within the lyrics of the famous Crosby, Stills, and Nash song "Wooden Ships," which say, "If you smile at me, I will understand. Because that is something everybody does in the same language."

A DANCE OF FEELINGS

The extremely important role that emotions play in our social interactions is the focus of psychologist and journalist Daniel Goleman's bestselling book, *Social Intelligence* (Bantam Books, 2006). In the following excerpt, Dr. Goleman describes what occurs in the brain during such interactions:

> We are wired to connect. Neuroscience has discovered that our brain's very design makes it sociable, inexorably drawn into an intimate brain-to-brain linkup whenever we engage with another person . . . During these neural linkups, our brains engage in an emotional tango, a dance of feelings . . . The resulting feelings have far-reaching consequences that ripple throughout our body, sending out cascades of hormones that regulate biological systems from our heart to our immune cells . . . That link is a double-edged sword: nourishing relationships have a beneficial impact on our health, while toxic ones can act like slow poison in our bodies.

If Goleman is correct, then we can begin to have a neurobiological understanding of why the quality of our relationships with family members, friends, work associates, and other important people in our lives strongly affects our general state of well-being.

This also tells us why having compassion for other people and engaging in acts of kindness makes us feel happy. It's because we are wired to respond that way. That these neurobiological connections would develop makes evolutionary sense, because being part of a social network can increase an individual's chance of survival.

CONSCIOUSNESS

Ever since I studied biology in college, I have been fascinated with the microbiology of how the body works. So, for me, trying to make a connection between meditation and the microbiology of how the mind works is a natural curiosity, particularly if it can help provide an understanding of the mechanisms for the healing power of meditation. This section will try to describe the neurobiological basis for consciousness. Later in the chapter is a description of what is happening in the brain during meditation. Then, I will review how the brain is able to acquire and preserve wisdom. The last section of this chapter will examine the neurobiological basis for the healing power of meditation.

New neuroscientific research that has been done in this field is very exciting, but it is also highly complex material. As V. S. Ramachandran, a neuroscientist at the Salk Institute and University of California at San Diego, says so simply in *A Brief Tour of Human Consciousness* (Pi Press, 2004), "The human brain . . . is the most complexly organized structure in the universe."

However, you should know that it is *not* necessary to understand the nature of consciousness at this level of detail to be able to practice and benefit from meditation. So it's okay to skip over portions of this chapter if you prefer not to get "bogged down" in these details. In fact, feel free to skip ahead to the last section, entitled "The Science of the Healing Power of Meditation," which summarizes many of the key concepts about the neurobiology of the way meditation works to heal illness and promote well-being. I would encourage you to refer frequently to Figure 6, Anatomy of the Brain on page 207 as you encounter references to the structures of the brain described here. One main "take-home lesson" I hope to convey is that the brain is not just an amorphous three and a half pounds of jelly-like homogenous tissue. Instead, the brain is composed of highly organized substructures, with different functions, that work together in an intricate and cooperative way to enable our minds to function.

STATES OF CONSCIOUSNESS

Our consciousness is sometimes likened to a movie of our lives playing in our head. But our consciousness is not really like a continuous movie. There does not appear to be a small group of neurons monitoring our lives like a homunculus in the center of our brains watching the movie. Instead, the feeling of consciousness is a thing of the whole experience. The visual images are often disjointed, fleeting, and symbolic, interspersed with sounds, phrases, thoughts, recollections, hopes, plans, and emotions. Underlying all of this is a basic awareness of being alive and conscious.

As a doctor, I have taken care of patients in many normal and pathological states of consciousness—sometimes all in the same patient. One recent case involved a retired U.S. Marine colonel who made an appointment to see me one month after he had fallen and hit the back of his head on the floor. His wife told me that, since his injury, he had been unable to maintain his balance. And, indeed, his examination showed he had difficulty standing, and his memory and speech were not quite normal. A brain scan done the same day showed that he had developed a large posttraumatic blood clot in his skull called a subdural hematoma. That large blood clot was compressing the right side of his brain, causing it to malfunction. He was immediately taken to surgery to evacuate the blood clot. But, by the next day, his level of consciousness was diminished, his left arm was weaker, and he was unable to swallow without choking. A repeat scan showed the blood clot had recurred, and he was again operated on to remove the new clot. However, the next postoperative brain scan showed he had begun to develop fluid collections on both sides of his brain.

Over the next couple of days, the old Marine colonel exhibited several different levels of consciousness that varied at different times: from being in a totally unresponsive deep coma; to a light coma with some awareness of his surroundings; to awake but only able to say one or two garbled words; to being agitated and thrashing about uncontrollably. Fortunately, with a lot of supportive care, he did finally mount a sustained recovery, including the return to a normal state of consciousness and his old amiable personality. After long-term physical therapy, he was able to walk and talk well.

WHAT IS CONSCIOUSNESS?

Exactly what constitutes consciousness varies from scientist to scientist. What follows is a review of how some leading neuroscientists are defining consciousness today. Then, I will offer my own definition of consciousness.

Gerald Edelman is a neurobiologist and Nobel laureate at the Scripps Research Institute in La Jolla, California, a nonprofit biomedical research organization. His book *Wider Than the Sky: The Phenomenal Gift of Consciousness* (Yale University Press, 2004) describes different levels of normal consciousness. There is "primary consciousness," which includes low-level awareness. And there are higher levels of consciousness that include interfacing with other elements in the brain such as language, bringing memory of past events to bear with concentrated awareness and attention.

Nobel Prize–winning DNA biophysicist Francis Crick (1916–2004) was a neuroscientist at the Salk Institute, also in La Jolla, when he wrote *The Astonishing Hypothesis: The Scientific Search for the Soul** (Scribner, 1994). In that book, Dr. Crick maintains that fellow neuroscientists basically agree on the following fundamental statements about consciousness:

- Not all the operations of the brain correspond to consciousness.

- Consciousness involves some form of memory, probably a very short-term one.

- Consciousness is closely associated with attention.

Crick adds that "what may prove difficult or impossible to establish are the details of the subjective nature of consciousness, since this may depend upon the exact symbolism employed by each conscious organism." This is an important point because it focuses on *why consciousness is a subjective experience.* Consciousness is not just a matter of sensory data in and action out. But it involves the subjective feelings that take place inside the conscious person.

The subjective nature of consciousness relates to the quality of feeling that a perception generates in an individual, or what are called "qualia." In *The Mind & the Brain* (HarperCollins, 2002), psychiatrist

---

Jeffrey Schwartz describes qualia as "[a] term many philosophers have adopted for the qualitative, raw, personal, subjective feel that we get from an experience or sensation. Every conscious state has a certain feel to it . . . not even the most detailed fMRI [functional magnetic resonance imaging] gives us more than the physical basis of perception or awareness; it doesn't come close to explaining what it feels like from the inside." And it is quite apparent that what conscious perceptions *feel like from the inside* varies a lot from person to person.

In the previously mentioned book *The Feeling of What Happens,* Damasio contends that there is a lot about consciousness that qualifies it to be a feeling. He also describes the important interaction that takes place between feelings and consciousness that governs our behavior and enables the expression of higher levels of thinking and consciousness. He writes,

> At first glance there is nothing distinctively human about emotions since it is clear that so many non-human creatures have emotions in abundance; and yet there is something quite distinctive about the way in which emotions have become connected to the complex ideas, values, principles, and judgments that only humans can have . . . It is through feelings, which are inwardly directed and private, that emotions, which are outwardly directed and public, begin their impact on the mind; *but the full and lasting impact of feelings requires consciousness,* because only along with the advent of a *sense of self* do feelings become known to the individual having them. [italics mine]

Consciousness as a "sense of a self" is a subject that interests neuroscientist V. S. Ramachandran. In *A Brief Tour of Human Consciousness,* he writes, "Far from being an epiphenomenon, the sense of self must have evolved through natural selection to enhance survival and, indeed, must include within it the ability to preserve its integrity and stability."

In order to survive, we must have the ability to consciously perceive what is going on around us. Our five senses give us that ability to perceive our surrounding environment by generating feelings in us about how that environment may be impacting our "self."

Dr. Edelman, mentioned earlier, describes consciousness as a "remembered present." In his book *Wider Than the Sky*, he describes the term in relation to his own state of conscious awareness:

> The scene is not just wider than the sky; it can contain many disparate elements—sensations, perceptions, images, memories, thoughts, emotions, aches, pains, vague feelings, and so on. Looked at from the inside, consciousness seems continually to change, yet at each moment it is all of a piece—what I have called "the remembered present"—reflecting the fact that all my past experiences engaged in forming my integrated awareness of this single moment.

Building on these foregoing ideas, I would propose the following as a concise definition of consciousness: Consciousness is a sense of self and one's surroundings in a remembered present. It is the connection of our emotions to our ideas, memories, values, principles, and judgments that gives us the feeling of the individuality of our consciousness, and the sense that we are a unique self, existing in a remembered present.

THE NEUROBIOLOGY OF CONSCIOUSNESS

Consciousness also has a physical component. The physiology of how the brain generates our sense of conscious awareness is described in some detail below.

Rocker-turned-neuroscientist Daniel Levitin, in *This Is Your Brain on Music* (Dutton, 2006), explains, "For cognitive scientists, the word *mind* refers to that part of each of us that embodies our thoughts, hopes, desires, memories, beliefs, and experiences. The brain, on the other hand, is an organ of the body, a collection of cells and water, chemicals and blood vessels that resides in the skull. Activity in the brain gives rise to the contents of the mind."

In the introduction to his book *The Astonishing Hypothesis,* Francis Crick put it this way: "The Astonishing Hypothesis is that You, your joys and your sorrows, your memories and your ambitions, your sense of personal identity and free will, are in fact no more than the behavior of a vast assembly of nerve cells and their associated molecules."

Many neuroscientists have been working to understand how consciousness works at the cellular and molecular level. It is amazing how much is becoming known. Hopefully, the details listed below will not be too daunting to follow.

Consciousness and Brain Wiring

Key parts of the brain create the feeling of consciousness. At the level of "brain wiring," consciousness depends on millions of reciprocal connections that cause reentrant, reverberating electrical circuits between the neurons (nerve cells) of the thalamus (located deep in the center of the brain) and the cerebral cortex (the gray matter in the furrowed outermost layer of the brain), the hippocampus, amygdala, anterior cingulate, and basal ganglia, with sensory input coming from the spinal cord.

When an electrochemical signal passes along the branches of a neuron, that signal must be able to be transmitted to the other neurons with which it connects. The tiny space between nerve cell connections is called a synapse. At the biochemical level, nerve cells in the brain communicate by releasing various specific chemicals, called neurotransmitters, which flow across the synapse to directly stimulate another neuron. Also, some neurotransmitter chemicals act by modifying the efficiency of signal transmission across the synapse. The chemical names of these neurotransmitter molecules are dopamine, serotonin, epinephrine, norepinephrine, acetylcholine, endorphins, and others. Not all neural circuits are stimulatory; some work by inhibition. When inhibitory neural circuits are not firing, "disinhibition" of other neurons occurs. (For example, disinhibition initiates bladder emptying.)

The ability of a person to consciously plan and imagine future actions is enabled by neural connections linking the brain's frontal lobes to and from the motor areas of the cerebral cortex, and coordination and sequencing of motor activity involving connections to and from the cerebellum. (See the brain diagram on page 207.)

It is clear from functional brain scans and EEG studies that when we plan or imagine an activity, the areas of the brain that become active are the same areas that are activated when we are really doing that activity.

As an example, if we are remembering a melody in our "mind's ear," or silently chanting a mantra, the same areas of the brain that process sound and control the motor area of the voice would be active. A similar phenomenon occurs when we observe someone else doing something. In response to seeing someone else perform an activity, our brain models, or mirrors, the activity just as if we were actually doing it ourselves. That's why, for instance, when we watch a ballplayer make a great play, or a dog sprint across a field, it makes us feel good. This is because it feels, in a way, like we did it, too!

Parallel processing of information signals, in different regions of the brain, allows the brain to perform several tasks at the same time. Thus, we are able to chew gum, walk, breathe, and think all at the same time. There are also so-called convergence zones in the brain that organize and sequence conscious thoughts and actions. This prevents the body from being pulled in different directions at the same time.

How a person actually comes to focus their awareness on a particular thing at any given time, and not on other things, has not yet been clarified by scientific research.

Memory

If consciousness is a sense of self in a remembered present, then the capacity to store and access memories is important for normal consciousness.

In order to store new memories, the brain requires the hippocampus (the seahorse-shaped structure deep in the sub-cortex of the brain) to be functioning well. The hippocampus is a structure that becomes damaged early in Alzheimer's disease patients, severely hampering their ability to form new memories.

Memories are stored diffusely throughout the cerebral cortex. And the memory of an activity or sensory image is stored near the area of the brain involved with the particular type of activity or sensation. For example, memories of visual images are stored near the visual cortex in the back of the brain, whereas memories of physical actions are stored near the motor cortex located near the top of the brain. This is why people with Alzheimer's disease have a variable degree of memory loss as the degenerative process "picks off" areas of memory in an uneven and unpredictable way in various parts of the brain.

A small area in the upper brain stem is also important to the formation of new memories. This area keeps a general level of arousal in the brain, which is necessary for the reverberating loops to continue long enough to help "solidify" a memory.

A patient that I evaluated in the emergency room and admitted to the hospital had an interesting memory disorder that illustrates the importance of the hippocampus to memory. Diane, a healthy fifty-year-old woman who had a long history of migraine headaches, came to the ER late one afternoon on a Mother's Day. Earlier that morning she had experienced one of her typical migraines. After awakening from an afternoon nap, she started asking her husband why there were bouquets of flowers in her room. She couldn't recall having received them from her daughters earlier that morning. Diane was extremely surprised to be told that it was Mother's Day, and scared that she couldn't remember anything she had done earlier that day. This condition is called transient global amnesia. Tests revealed she had a normal electroencephalogram (EEG) and MRI brain scan. Her neurologic physical exam, performed by myself and a consulting neurologist, was normal. Our best guess (although not proven) was that Diane's migraine earlier that day had triggered a brief interruption of blood flow to her hippocampus, temporarily blocking her ability to form new memories. Twenty-four hours later her capacity to store new memories returned to normal. But, Diane never recovered her memory for those Mother's Day events.

Left Brain/Right Brain

It used to be said that humans use only a small portion of their brain's capacity. But we now know that this is not the case. The brain is an organ made of only a little more than three pounds of jelly-like tissue. In order to perform all the millions of amazing tasks it does, the brain is organized in such a way that almost all its capacity is available to be utilized.

Human brains have evolved a capacity to make more efficient use of available brain power (neuronal mass) by localizing certain functions to the left or right side. Language capacity, for example, is localized mostly on the left. Creative problem solving and spatial-temporal reasoning is localized more on the right side of the brain.

In *The Wisdom Paradox* (Gotham, 2005), neuropsychologist Elkhonon Goldberg presents recent experimental data concerning other ways the two halves of the brain differ. Structural differences between the two sides of the brain include far more spindle cells (a specialized type of neuron) on the right side of the brain. These spindle cells are very long and are thought to allow areas of the brain that are far apart to communicate. The large number of these spindle cells on the right side of the brain may allow better communication between different brain areas, as might be necessary for creative problem solving.

PET and fMRI scans allow us to see which areas of the brain become active during problem solving and accessing stored information. Functionally, it seems that the right half of the brain dominates in the processing of new, unfamiliar information and situations that require creative problem solving. Later, this newly processed information becomes more encoded in patterns that are stored in the left side of the brain. When we are involved in a familiar task, the mind can quickly access these patterns on the left. This enables the left side of the brain to be more involved in pattern recognition dealing with well-established cognitive skills, like language.

In his book, Dr. Goldberg describes experimental data that shows what he calls a kind of "right-to-left shift of the 'center of cognitive gravity' throughout the lifespan of a person . . . The right hemisphere is of foremost importance in our youth, the season of daring, of navigating uncharted waters. The left hemisphere is of foremost importance in mature years, the season of wisdom, of seeing new things through the prism of vast past experience."

I have noticed this type of cognitive shift in my own life. When I was young, I spent a couple of summers hitchhiking around the United States, something I would never do now. I didn't know then that my hitchhiking adventures were motivated by right-brain activity, or that much of the wisdom I would rely on to guide my actions later would require more left-brain activity.

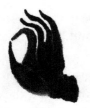

THE NEUROBIOLOGY
OF MEDITATION

Based on the type of neuroscientific research studies cited earlier, we can begin to put together a partial understanding of what is going on inside the brain during meditation.

The general activity of the brain's frontal lobes, which are involved with complex planning and decision making, has been found to be diminished during meditation. This is consistent with the knowledge that, during meditation, thinking is diminished. Also diminished is activity in the parietal lobes. This area of the brain controls motor and sensory function. It makes sense that during sitting meditation this area would be less active, because your muscles are not moving much and the overall amount of sensory input is also reduced. This would naturally result in less sensory and motor input to one of the brain's main connection centers called the thalamus. And, indeed, activity in the thalamus is reduced during meditation.

One region of the brain that becomes more active during meditation is a specific area called the left prefrontal cortex, an area of brain located at the "front" pole of the left frontal lobe, just behind our forehead. (The line on the brain diagram on page 207 pointing to the frontal lobe cortex is also pointing to the area of the prefrontal cortex.) Increased activity in this area has been correlated with increased feelings of happiness and compassion. Portions of the limbic system, deep within the brain, that generate our emotional responses become more active during meditation. The brain waves, as measured with scalp electrodes attached to an EEG machine, show a shift away from the predominant beta waves of aroused, conscious thought toward more theta waves. Theta waves have been associated with a feeling of calm contentment and deep relaxation.

Which group of neurons initiates and controls the shift in the above parameters, away from normal consciousness to the meditation mode of consciousness, is unknown. But we can begin the process just by willing ourselves to attend to a meditation focal point, like the breath or a mantra. The more we practice meditation, the more "wired" our neural pathways become to quickly and efficiently achieve a meditative state of consciousness. (More on this on page 223 in the section "Neurons That Fire Together Wire Together.")

The neurology of how we cultivate insight (wisdom) by practicing meditation is also speculative at this time. In the next section, "Learning and Wisdom," I'll review Dr. Goldberg's contention that much of wisdom is stored in patterns in the left side of our cerebral cortex. It is possible that stimulating the left prefrontal cortex, as occurs in meditation, might trigger some associations that connect together in novel ways patterns stored elsewhere in the left cerebral cortex, producing a conscious insight.

BEHAVIOR

We all exhibit patterns of mental and physical behaviors that are mediated by inherited, hard-wired groups of neurons that have become modified by previous experience. These behaviors may include the capacity for anger, hatred, jealousy, fear, and other "negative seeds," as well as "positive seeds" of joy, compassion, peace, and love. These behaviors may be orchestrated intentionally or generated automatically after being prompted by a stimulus of a perception or a thought.

We will likely never know what another person's consciousness feels like, or even be able to know what someone else is thinking from an external analysis of neurological activity. But knowing how *our own brain* and consciousness works on a neurological level may help us learn to modify the behavior of our own conscious and unconscious processes for the better.

I have seen this work in patients who have taken meditation classes. Many of these people have successfully reduced their symptoms of stress or illness by meditating. They learn to direct their consciousness away from compulsive overthinking or overreacting, toward a more present-oriented, peaceful awareness and mindfulness of action.

Our conscious actions may also be informed and modified by our accumulated wisdom. Bringing wisdom to bear can influence how frequently certain negative behaviors and negative mental states manifest in us, and how to skillfully deal with them (by using meditation and other means) when they are present. The next section will discuss the neurobiology of how we acquire wisdom.

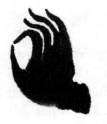

LEARNING AND WISDOM

What we learn over the course of our lifetime has a powerful impact on our physical health. Learning healthy habits, such as engaging in regular physical exercise, eating nutritious foods, avoiding intake of toxins, making use of basic medical knowledge, and learning how to connect well with other people, all have a potential impact on our health and longevity. Meditation, in addition to being an intrinsically healthy state of being, can also help us gain wisdom about what actions and behaviors are healthy. The neurobiology of how we learn and acquire wisdom, how wisdom is stored for future use, and how meditation can enhance this process are the subjects of this section.

LEARNING

Beyond childhood, adult human brains retain their capacity to develop and change, mostly on the basis of modifying existing neural connections, and partly on the basis of growing new nerve cells. These new neurons form from neural stem cells lining the ventricles of the brain, and then migrate to areas of increased cognitive activity.

When learning takes place, what is happening in the brain at the cellular level? In his book *Synaptic Self: How Our Brains Become Who We Are* (Penguin, 2003), neuropsychologist Joseph LeDoux states that learning takes place when synapses in the brain are physiologically modified on the basis of an experience and the parallel association of that experience with various perceptual inputs (sensory, auditory, visual, and so on).

Emotions and feelings also play an important role in learning. Our emotions, and the feelings they induce, interact with our consciousness to make us aware of the feeling of what is happening. These feelings help us learn how to best respond to rapidly changing life situations. And, learning takes place when the conscious mind brings memory and internalized values and principles into the mix. We can then learn to modify future behaviors and reactions for the better.

Look again at the brain diagram on page 207. One anatomical clue that demonstrates how closely the emotions and memory are tied together in the learning process is that the hippocampus (a structure vital for forming new memories) lies anatomically adjacent to the amygdala, which is responsible for triggering some of our strongest emotions. Memories are most permanently stored in our brains when they are formed at the same time that a strong emotional reaction has occurred. Since memory is tied to our ability to learn, the things we learn the easiest are the things that have had the most emotional impact on us.

Neurons That Fire Together Wire Together

Neuroscientists like Joseph LeDoux and Gerald Edelman have advanced the theory that "neurons that fire together wire together." This means that when a group of neurons is activated by the "firing" of an electrochemical signal across their synapses, this produces changes that "wire" the neurons together in a closer grouping by increasing the number and efficiency of synaptic ties between those neurons.

Buddhism talks about "seeds," such as anger, fear, and happiness, which are said to be contained in our "store consciousness." These seeds are groups of neural pathways that fire together based on genetically determined brain-wiring patterns, which can be modified by past experience. In other words, these groups of neurons have become "wired together." When we are stimulated by new encounters or thoughts, these coordinated neural responses manifest in us. But, they seem to produce a mental and physical reaction, or pattern of behavior, that often feels familiar and repetitive.

It is likely that we codify the knowledge that comes from experience in the form of neural networks that become bound together in a pattern. This binding together occurs as a result of a group of neurons that are stimulated to fire at the same time. At first, this produces very temporary changes in the state of the neurons and synapses involved. But, with repetition, more permanent changes occur. These changes include increases in the number of dendrite connections (branches) between these neurons and improved efficiency of synaptic transmission within the neural group. Also, nearby other noninvolved neural connections are pruned or just wither away as the brain develops and evolves. Together, these changes produce a phenomenon in which stimulation of only part of the neural network will cause all of the previously bundled neurons to fire, producing a recognizable pattern.

Neuroplasticity

The functional capacity of our brains is strongly affected by the ways neurons can change and become organized into new groupings. This phenomenon is called neuroplasticiy. One of the best books written on the subject of neuroplasticity is *The Mind and the Brain: Neuroplasticity and the Power of Mental Force* by Jeffrey Schwartz, MD. His book reviews some fascinating research studies that investigate a variety of forms of neuroplasticity. A few of these experimental studies are summarized below.

One such groundbreaking study was done way back in 1923 by Karl Lashley, a pioneer in the field of neuropsychology. He plotted movement maps of the brain of a monkey by directly stimulating with electrodes different spots in the motor cortex of the brain and then observing which muscle twitched. Dr. Lashley plotted four movement maps in the same rhesus monkey over the course of a month. To his surprise, he found each map was significantly different from the previous map, and the differences became progressively greater in the later maps. Dr. Lashley theorized these differences reflected changes in neural control of muscles that were based on experience or use over time. He concluded that muscles that move more receive a greater cortical representation than muscles that move less.

Many years later, this conclusion was reinforced by experiments neuroscientist Randolph Nudo performed on squirrel monkeys, which were published in 1996 in the *Journal of Neuroscience*. Dr. Nudo plotted movement maps of the monkey's forearm, wrist, and fingers. Then he taught them, over the course of weeks, to retrieve small food pellets from a tiny dispenser, which required them to learn to manipulate their fingers with great dexterity. After they learned this skill, he again plotted movement maps of their arms and fingers. Dr. Nudo found that there was a "dramatic remodeling of the monkeys' motor cortices. The area that became active when a monkey moved his digits, wrist, and forearm had doubled . . . The neurons controlling the busy fingers had undergone the neural equivalent of suburban sprawl, colonizing more space in the motor cortex, crowding out neurons that controlled some other part of the body (though with no obvious effect on other body parts)."

Another example of neural rezoning in response to a learned behavior can be found in the 1995 experiments of behavioral neuroscientist Edward Taub and neuropsychologist Thomas Elbert. They studied the sensory maps of six violinists, two cello players, and a guitarist, and compared them to those of nonmusicians. Light pressure was applied to their fingers and magnetic EEGs recorded the neural activity in their sensory cortex. All the volunteers were right-handed, but the musicians had developed a high degree of dexterity in the fingers of their left hand needed to perform the complex fingering patterns along the frets of the stringed instruments. (The right-hand movements necessary to play these string instruments are much simpler.) What the study found was that compared to nonmusicians, the amount of cerebral cortex that corresponded to the left-hand fingers was much greater in the musicians. There was no difference between the groups in the cortical representation in the right-hand fingers.

In 1995, Cornelius Weiller, a professor of neurology in Germany, studied another type of neuroplasticity in six men who had experienced a severe left-brain stroke. This caused them to be unable to speak, because the stroke had destroyed their speech area, called Wernike's area. Later, these men eventually regained their ability to speak. PET scans were then done while these men performed word exercises. The scans showed that "regions in the right hemisphere, corresponding in position to the left cortex's Wernike's area and other language centers, became active. Recovery, it seemed, had been accompanied by cortical reorganization. Right-brain areas analogous to the left brain's damaged zones had taken over their function."

Research studies like those mentioned above led Dr. Schwartz to write, "The neuroplasticity I am talking about extends beyond the formation of a synapse here, the withering away of a synapse there. It refers to the wholesale remapping of neural real estate . . . It is the neural version of suburban sprawl: real estate that used to serve one purpose being developed for another."

The flip side of neuroplasticity is that it can sometimes harm us. For instance, exposing oneself to repetitive doses of toxic media, such as viewing many movies that contain gratuitous violence or sex, can rewire the brain in such a way that might later predispose one to adverse behavior. Also a chronic pain syndrome can be self-reinforcing if the brain pathways become rewired in such a way that causes an increased perception of pain.

Neuroplasticity adversely affecting the brain's control of motor function might also explain the abnormally tentative walking style seen in many elderly people. Schwartz postulates that

> With age, walking becomes more fraught with the risk of a spill, so many people begin to walk in an ever-more constrained way. Old people become erect and stiff, or stooped, using shorter steps and a slower pace. As a result, they get less "practice" at confidant striding —bad idea. Because they no longer walk normally and instead "over-practice" a rigid shuffling gait, the motor cortex of fluid movement degrades . . . The result: we burn a trace of the old-folks' walk into our brain, eventually losing the ability to walk as we once did . . . There is, though, a bright side: there is every reason to believe that practicing normal movements with careful guided exercise may help prevent, or even reverse, the maladaptive changes.

The Brain That Changes Itself by Norman Doidge, MD, is another excellent book that reports on recent research investigating neuroplasticity of the brain. Dr. Doidge describes some elegant experiments that map the brain using a new noninvasive technique called transcranial magnetic stimulation, or TMS. This technique employs a magnetic field that can be aimed at a small group of neurons in the motor cortex of the brain, for example, causing them to fire an electrochemical signal that is transmitted to other neurons. Then the researchers look to see which muscles are stimulated to contract. Because it is painless and harmless, humans can be studied repeatedly, thereby mapping changes in the motor cortex over time.

One clinical investigation in the early 1990s by Dr. Alvaro Pascual-Leone's group at Beth Israel Deaconess Medical Center in Boston used TMS to study a group of blind people learning to read Braille. It was found that the brain map for their Braille-reading index finger took up a larger area of brain than the index fingers of non-Braille readers. As these students continued learning to read Braille, it was found that after just a few days of practice the area of their brain devoted to their index finger further expanded. The speed of these changes of neuroplasticity was truly astounding. And after a couple of days of not practicing, the area of brain devoted to the Braille-reading index finger diminished.

Similar changes in brain mapping would likely explain why musicians (like fellow trumpet players) often notice their playing ability diminishes after just a couple days of not practicing their instrument. Fortunately, the losses are easily restored with practice, which speaks to another phenomenon about learning: there is a difference between short-term learning gains versus long-term learning gains. The structural and chemical changes that account for these long-term learning gains are a subject of ongoing scientific investigation.

The Brain That Changes Itself also reports some other interesting experiments by Dr. Pascual-Leone using TMS brain mapping to study sighted people who were blindfolded for several days. The visual cortex is located in a totally different area of the brain than the brain's sensory and auditory cortex. But, in the blindfolded people, it was found that, after as few as two days, the unused area of brain that normally processes visual information began to process the sense of touch coming from their hands and auditory information coming from their ears. So the brain was reorganizing itself in just a few days! This explains how blind people can develop exquisite senses of touch and hearing that help them compensate for their disability.

First Experiences Become the Model

Humans often learn by mirroring what they see. Put simply: monkey see, monkey do. And as we learn, our synaptic connections become modified as described above, and even new neurons can likely be acquired. This brain plasticity explains why our early experiences have a profound effect on how we react to situations later. This is because the early experiences have caused changes in the wiring patterns of our brain, which then affects the way we process the later experiences. These changes are most profound in early life when new neural connections are naturally being formed at a rapid rate.

This phenomenon highlights the importance of our early relationships with people like parents, siblings, and mentors. These early experiences will form the basis of how we learn to interact with other people later. For more on this topic, see the *Time* magazine cover story entitled "The New Science of Siblings: How Your Siblings Make You Who You Are" (July 10, 2006).

WISDOM

The acquisition of wisdom is fundamentally a very important type of learning. My good friend, Greg O'Leary, once defined wisdom as "good judgment informed by experience." All of us—not just so-called wise men—have the capacity to gain and retain insights and wisdom. (But, wise men probably accumulate a larger amount of wisdom over their lifetime.)

In *The Wisdom Paradox,* Dr. Goldberg (mentioned earlier in the chapter) explains how previously stored memories, and the recognition of other stored mental patterns, are integrated by the frontal lobes of the brain in the development of wisdom. Goldberg writes,

> Throughout history, wisdom has been understood as the fusion of the intellectual and moral, spiritual and practical dimensions . . . According to many definitions, wisdom implies the ability to integrate pragmatic "actor-centered" and ethical "empathy-driven" considerations . . . The unique role of the prefrontal cortex lies in its providing the neural machinery for bringing these two factors together in a single well-integrated decision-making process . . . It is the frontal lobes that organize our mental skills into complex ensembles. The frontal lobes are in charge of making plans, of charting paths that the organism must take in solving a wide range of problems. Like the conductor pointing his or her baton at various members of the orchestra as the music unfolds, the frontal lobes call upon specific mental skills and abilities and weave them into complex behaviors.

From an evolutionary standpoint, acquiring language was also key to mankind's ability to develop and store complex ideas and wisdom. In *Wider Than the Sky,* Dr. Edelman writes that higher-order consciousness "requires semantic ability, that is, the assignment of meaning to a symbol. In its most developed form, it requires linguistic ability, that is, the mastery of a whole system of symbols and a grammar."

Language is one of the most powerful tools we have to place into symbolic patterns the accumulated wisdom that we learn from outside sources and from our own life experience. Using language, we can easily and efficiently access this information in the future so we can consciously communicate it to ourselves, as well as transmit it to other people, and even pass the knowledge down through the generations as a kind of accumulated "wisdom of the ages" that is part of the cultural evolution of our species.

Wisdom and the Aging Brain

In very advanced age, brain atrophy and neural degenerative changes occur that can lead to what doctors call mild cognitive impairment (MCI) or the dementia of Alzheimer's disease (for more on these conditions, see Chapter 2). I have seen Alzheimer's disease lead to dreadfully serious health consequences, like accidental falls causing hip or skull fractures, malnutrition, urinary incontinence and infection, ill health due to failure to take prescribed medication or taking the medication incorrectly, or failure to seek appropriate medical attention when symptoms of a serious illness arise. And, indeed, Alzheimer's disease is a well-recognized cause of death.

As they begin to experience a decline in their cognitive function, one issue that will confront many older people is this: how they can store, retain access to, and even expand their accumulated wisdom, despite the degeneration of neurologic pathways that occurs in advanced age. Are there any strategies that can optimize their ability to attain new insights, and continue to make use of the wisdom they have acquired? The answer is yes. There is evidence that if people make a practice of continuing to engage in vigorous cognitive and physical activity throughout life, this can result in increased neural mass and more neural connections in some areas of the brain. If a person develops a larger number of neurons and neural connections, this can then diminish the effect of the age-related degenerative changes that can cause cognitive decline in old age. In people with early Alzheimer's disease, this could also potentially slow the development of more advanced symptoms of dementia.

Doing crossword puzzles and sudoku, or playing games like bridge or chess, can help elderly people remain mentally bright, because of the way these activities strengthen and increase neural connections. Also, it appears that, rather than just engaging in familiar activities that one is already good at doing, trying new challenges and learning new skills are even more potent behaviors for slowing the decline of brain function in old age.

Other exercises for improving the functioning of an older brain are described in the book *Mozart's Brain and the Fighter Pilot: Unleashing Your Brain's Potential* (Three Rivers Press, 2002) by Richard Restak, MD. Also, the Posit Science "Brain Fitness Program" provides a series of exercises developed by neuroscientists and psychologists (see www.posit science.com).

Regular physical activity can also slow mental decline. Researchers at the Harvard School of Public Health found that simply walking two or three hours a week increases cognition and memory in elderly women. Research has shown that physical exercise acts as an important stimulus for the brain to produce the new neurons that migrate from deep in the ventricles to other brain areas. So, exercising your body helps build up your brain!

Meditation is yet another way elderly people can improve their mental capacity. Meditation helps people acquire new insights and improves their flexibility of mind and ability to concentrate. This enhanced ability to concentrate enables elderly people to preserve their capacity to learn. For elderly people who are still able to walk, walking meditation is an ideal practice. This is because it combines meditation with the activity of walking, which has been proven to improve cognitive function.

In *The Wisdom Paradox,* Dr. Goldberg makes the point that with advanced age there occurs an inevitable decline in the ability to form *new* memories. This occurs because the hippocampus, which is so important to the machinery of forming new memories, is particularly sensitive to the degenerative effects of the general neural decline that accompanies old age. However, since previously formed *old* memories and other brain patterns are diffusely stored in many locations throughout the cerebral cortex, they are much more resistant to decline with advancing age. So, older people usually retain the ability to access previously stored memories of past experiences and memories of solutions to past problems.

Goldberg contends that much of our accumulated wisdom depends, not so much on an ongoing reasoning process, but more on recognizing life patterns that are similar to previously stored mental patterns that we can then apply to new life situations. He explains,

> With age, the number of real-life cognitive tasks requiring a painfully effortful, deliberate creation of new mental constructs seems to be diminishing. Instead, problem-solving (in the broadest sense) takes increasingly the form of pattern recognition. This means that with age we accumulate an increasing number of cognitive templates. Consequently, a growing number of future cognitive challenges is increasingly likely to be relatively readily covered by a preexisting template, or will require only a slight modification of a previously formed mental template. Increasingly, decision-making takes the form of pattern recognition rather than of problem-solving.

Therefore, the essence of our wisdom is encoded in these patterns, or "cognitive templates," stored in our brain. Most elderly people can usually still access these patterns, despite having some memory impairment and mild cognitive decline.

So the good news is that, if we remain relatively healthy and mentally active, we can retain much of our capacity for awareness of accumulated wisdom well into our advanced years.

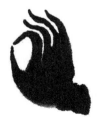

THE SCIENCE OF THE HEALING POWER OF MEDITATION

Meditation is not new. It has been practiced by many diverse traditions for thousands of years because countless millions of people have found the practice beneficial. Whether we are talking about meditation as practiced within the tradition of Buddhism, Hinduism, or Taoism, or forms of meditation that have been practiced within the Jewish and Christian traditions, or forms of movement meditation like t'ai chi, yoga, and qi gong, or what contemporary spiritual advisor Eckhart Tolle calls "the power of now," or what Ram Dass calls "the process of calming and centering"—these are all paths that can potentially allow the individual to benefit from the healing power of meditation.

This chapter has reviewed the science of how the mind and brain function. Neuroscientists are just now beginning to understand how meditation works and what it is about meditation that gives it the power to heal illness and promote wellness.

Research studies reviewed earlier in this chapter have shown that the connections between neurons in the brain, and even the very functions of whole areas of the brain, are in a constant state of change. Brain mapping has shown that when we repetitively practice an activity the amount of brain tissue devoted to the activity expands, and even other distant areas of the brain can become recruited to aid in the activity. It is also clear that when the mind practices an activity, certain neurological pathways are reinforced and "wired together."

Similar changes must occur in the brain as a result of practicing meditation. This helps explain why the more we practice meditation the easier it becomes to achieve the meditative state of consciousness. It's because the brain pathways for meditation become progressively more "wired" together and likely recruit a larger area of brain "real estate" into the process of meditation. So, with practice, it becomes progressively easier to "trigger" the meditative state and enter into deep meditation.

As discussed in Chapter 2, medical research has found that happy people derive a health benefit and actually live longer than people who are generally unhappy. Healthy emotional responses to meditation, such as happiness, are self-reinforcing in that the more time we spend dwelling in happiness the more we are "wired" to achieve the state of happiness. Conversely, the less time we spend dwelling in negative states like sadness, fear, and anger, the less those brain pathways are reinforced, and those negative states become less likely to be triggered by events. This explains, on a neurological basis, the validity of Spinoza's philosophical advice that humans should endeavor to frequently expose themselves to stimuli that trigger positive nourishing emotions as a way of avoiding dwelling in negativity. The Zen perspective calls this "watering the good seeds."

During meditation, blood flow and metabolism are increased in areas of the brain that are known to be associated with feelings of happiness and well-being, like the left prefrontal cortex and the limbic system. This phenomenon is partly mediated by the neurons releasing a neurotransmitter called dopamine, which has been correlated with a feeling of happiness. And the neurons can release molecules called endorphins, which reduce pain and produce a feeling of satisfaction.

Meditation also helps people feel happier by reducing the neurohormonal response to stress and assuaging the emotions of fear and anger. By practicing meditation we learn to decrease our obsessive thinking. We can then avoid dwelling in painful regret about past events and reduce our worrying about future events. This diminishes our chance of developing depression or chronic anxiety. And, as we have seen in Chapter 2, reducing stress, anxiety, and depression has a positive impact on our physical health and longevity.

It seems quite likely that any neural stimulation that occurs in a repetitive fashion has the capacity to cause the eventual "remapping of neural real estate." Repetition of thought patterns probably function this way as well. One can reinforce a concept, such as impermanence, interconnectedness, or compassion, by repetitively chanting or meditating on a spiritual poem, like "The Five Insights" or "Watering the Seeds." These practices would be expected to cause a rewiring or remolding of the neural pathways in the brain. The effect of these newly rewired neural pathways would be to keep these concepts alive in us and reverberating as constant insights. These insights can affect our behavior in ways that not only benefit other people with whom we are interconnected, but also result in us feeling happier and living longer.

Meditation can cause neuroplastic changes in the brain that modify the way pain signals (from a chronically painful part of the body) are processed by the brain, in such a way that the perception of pain is reduced. Meditation can also cause the release of endorphins, which reduce pain perception. Using meditation to control pain (see "Meditations for Transforming Pain" in Chapter 4) can improve quality of life, whether a person is suffering chronic pain caused by arthritis, cancer, fibromyalgia, irritable bowel syndrome, neuropathy, or some other chronic painful condition.

The capacity of the brain's neurons to change and reorganize themselves—called neuroplasticity—may explain why the modeling meditation exercise described in Chapter 4 works to decrease pain. This technique describes modeling the painful body part after the same part of the body on the opposite side that is functioning well. Through repetition, this modeling technique might eventually cause a physical remodeling and rewiring of motor and sensory neurons on the affected side of the brain, allowing the painful body part to function more normally and with less pain.

The brain has many connections via the nervous system to the heart and blood vessels, so it should be no surprise that meditation has the capacity to lower heart rate and blood pressure, which are potentially heart-healthy effects. Indeed, one clinical trial (reviewed in Chapter 2) found that people with congestive heart failure who meditate had improved exercise capacity.

Medical research has found strong links between the nervous system and the immune system. This may eventually explain why meditation has been proven to improve aspects of the immune system that may help us fight or prevent cancer and infection.

Brain scans have demonstrated that during meditation the thinking and planning parts of the brain become relatively metabolically inactive. So, people who suffer from insomnia due to being unable to turn off their thoughts at night can successfully use meditation techniques to get to sleep (see "Meditations for a Good Night's Sleep" in Chapter 4).

Many other potential health benefits of meditation were described in Chapter 2, along with references to the medical studies that have shown meditation to be of clinical efficacy. The exact mechanism by which meditation produces its beneficial effects in some of these illnesses has yet to be determined. These health benefits include using meditation to treat psoriasis, obesity, and chronic fatigue; to diminish symptoms of asthma, chronic lung disease, PMS, and hot flashes associated with menopause; to prevent stomach ulcers and heartburn that can be caused by stress-induced hyperacidity of the stomach; to reduce the frequency of migraine and tension headaches; to relieve the emotional distress of anxiety, sadness, and minor depression; and to help people with mild cognitive impairment and Alzheimer's disease improve their concentration and flexibility of mind.

Meditation exercises, like Buddha's Breathing Exercises and Meditation on the Whole Person, make us more aware of our inner feelings. This allows us to better assess whether our bodies are in a state of distress or ill health and if corrective action needs to be taken. Meditation may give us healthy insights that modify our behavior so we may start to exercise more, eat healthier foods, and avoid exposure to toxins.

During meditation, spontaneous insights occur that can change our behavior for the better and allow us to respond to life's problems more skillfully. Meditation insights can allow us to connect and communicate better with our family members, friends, work associates, and other people in our community, so we can collectively help each other to survive and thrive. By meditating, we can learn to respond to negative situations that we experience with a greater sense of acceptance and peace. We can begin to derive happiness from the appreciation of simple ordinary things such as taking a walk or seeing a colorful patch of wild flowers on a green hill against a deep blue sky.

These are the many ways and means by which meditation can contribute to your better health and well-being. Understanding and applying the healing practice of meditation truly constitutes a science of body and mind.

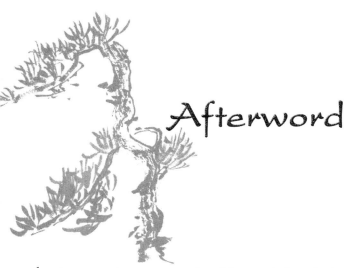

Afterword

In the preceding pages, what I have tried to do is teach meditation, and describe how meditation can help heal illness and promote wellness.

This book also represents a quest to develop a philosophy about the human condition within nature that is all of one piece. I am motivated by a desire to identify my own core values, and then try to live by those principles. Those principles blend insights drawn from both Eastern Zen and Western scientific traditions.

It is in the spirit of compassion that I offer this book and these humble thoughts to you, dear reader. No view is the absolute truth, and no words can resolve all the contradictions. The validation of whether meditation works is not in the discussion, but in the practice.

—Gabriel Weiss

Mindfulness Bibliography

Articles

Arias et al. "Systematic review of meditation techniques as treatments for medical illness." *Journal of Alternative and Complementary Medicine* 2006; 12(8): 817.

Bakke et al. "The effect of hypnotic-guided imagery on psychological well-being and immune function in patients with prior breast cancer." *Journal of Psychosomatic Research* 2002; 53: 1131–37.

Barnes et al. "Impact of meditation on resting and ambulatory blood pressure and heart rate in youth." *Psychosomatic Medicine* 2004 Nov–Dec; 66(6): 909.

Benson et al. "Decreased premature ventricular contractions through the use of the relaxation response in patients with stable ischaemic heart disease." *Lancet* 1975 Aug 30; 2(7931): 380–82.

———. "The relaxation response." *Psychiatry* 1974 Feb; 37(1): 37.

Bormann et al. "Effects of spiritual mantra repetition on HIV outcomes: a randomized clinical trial." *Journal of Behavioral Medicine* 2006 Aug; 29(4): 359.

"The Brain: A User's Guide." *Time* magazine cover story, January 29, 2007.

Bruya, B. "Going to Pieces with Mark Epstein" (interview for Amazon.com). http://human-nature.com/interviews/epstein.html.

Butts and Sternberg. "Neuroendocrine factors alter host defense by modulating immune function." *Cellular Immunology* 2008 Mar 6.

Canter. "The therapeutic effects of meditation." *British Medical Journal* 2003; 326: 1049.

Carlson et al. "Mindfulness-based stress reduction in relation to quality of life, mood, symptoms of stress, and immune parameters in breast and prostate cancer outpatients." *Psychosomatic Medicine* 2003 Jul–Aug; 65(4): 571.

Cohen-Katz et al. "The effects of mindfulness-based stress reduction on nurse stress and burnout." *Holistic Nursing Practice* 2005 Mar–Apr: 78.

Curiati et al. "Meditation reduces sympathetic activation and improves the quality of life in elderly patients with optimally controlled heart failure: a prospective randomized study." *Journal of Alternative and Complementary Medicine* 2005 Jun; 11(3): 465.

Danner, et al. "Positive emotions in early life and longevity: findings from the nun study." *Journal of Personality and Social Psychology* 2001 May; 80(5): 804–13.

Davidson, and Kabat-Zinn. "Alterations in brain and immune function produced by mindfulness meditation." *Psychosomatic Medicine* 2003 Jul–Aug; 64(4): 564.

Ekman. "Facial Expressions of Emotion: New Findings, New Questions." *Psychological Science* 3 (1992): 34–38.

Ganguli, et al. "Rates and predictors of mortality in an aging, rural, community-based cohort: the role of depression." *Archives of General Psychiatry* 2002 Nov; 59(11): 1046–52.

Gazella. "Bringing mindfulness to medicine: an interview with Jon Kabat-Zinn, Ph.D." *Advances in Mind-Body Medicine* 2005, Summer; 21(2): 22–27.

Gilad, G.M., and V.H. Gilad. "Strain, stress, neurodegeneration and longevity." *Mechanisms of Ageing and Development* 1995 Mar; 78(2): 75–83.

Gilray, et al. "Dispositional optimism and all-cause and cardiovascular mortality in a prospective cohort of elderly Dutch men and women." *Archives of General Psychiatry* 2004 Nov; 61: 1126–35.

Goodale, Domar, and Benson. "Alleviation of premenstrual syndrome symptoms with the relaxation response." *Obstetrics and Gynecology* 1990 Apr; 75(4): 649.

Hentoff. "Final Chorus, Louis Armstrong: Music Heals." *JazzTimes.com* 2006 Dec.

Hershberger. "Prescribing happiness: positive psychology and family medicine." *Family Medicine* 2005 Oct; 37(9): 630–34.

Irvin et al. "The effects of relaxation training on menopausal symptoms." *Journal of Psychsomatic Obstetrics & Gynecology* 1996 Dec; 17(4): 202.

Iwasa et al. "Subjective well-being and all-cause mortality among middle-aged and elderly people living in an urban Japanese community." *Nippon Ronen Igakkai Zasshi (Japanese Journal of Geriatrics)* 2005 Nov; 42(6): 677–83.

Iyer, Pico. "The Dalai Lama's Journey." *Time* magazine, March 31, 2008.

Jacobs et al. "Multifactor behavioral treatment of chronic sleep-onset insomnia using stimulus control and the relaxation response: a preliminary study." *Behavior Modification* 1993 Oct; 17(4): 498.

Jain et al. "A randomized controlled trial of mindfulness meditation versus relaxation training: effects on distress, positive states of mind, rumination, and distraction." *Annals of Behavioral Medicine* 2007 Feb; 33(1): 11.

Jayadevappa et al. "Effectiveness of transcendental meditation on functional capacity and quality of life of African Americans with congestive heart failure: a randomized control study." *Ethnicity and Disease* 2007 Winter; 17(1): 172.

Kabat-Zinn et al. "Effectiveness of a meditation-based stress reduction program in the treatment of anxiety disorders." *American Journal of Psychiatry* 1992 Jul; 149(7): 936.

————. "Influence of a mindfulness meditation-based stress reduction intervention on rates of skin clearing in patients with moderate to severe psoriasis undergoing phototherapy (UVB) and photochemotherapy." *Psychosomatic Medicine* 1998 Sep–Oct; 60(5): 625.

Kaplan et al. "The impact of a meditation-based stress reduction program on fibromyalgia." *General Hospital Psychiatry* 1993 Sep; 15(5): 284.

Keefer et al. "A one-year follow-up of relaxation response meditation as a treatment for irritable bowel syndrome." *Behaviour Research and Therapy* 2002 May; 40(5): 541.

————. "The effects of relaxation response meditation on the symptoms of irritable bowel syndrome: results of a controlled treatment study." *Behaviour Research and Therapy* 2001 Jul; 39(7): 801.

Lane et al. "Brief meditation training can improve perceived stress and negative mood." *Alternative Therapies in Health and Medicine* 2007 Jan–Feb; 13(1): 38.

Lengacher et al. "Immune responses to guided imagery during breast cancer treatment." *Biological Research for Nursing* 2008 Jan; 9(3): 205–14.

Leserman et al. "The efficacy of the relaxation response in preparing for cardiac surgery." *Behavioral Medicine* 1989 Fall; 15(3): 111–17.

Levy et al. "Longevity increased by positive self-perceptions of aging." *Journal of Personality and Social Psychology* 2002; 83(2): 261–70.

Manocha et al. "Sahaja yoga in the management of moderate to severe asthma: a randomized controlled trial." *Thorax* 2002 Feb; 57(2): 110.

Maruta et al. "Optimists vs pessimists: survival rate among medical patients over a 30-year period." *Mayo Clinic Proceedings* 2000 Feb; 75(2): 140–43.

McDonald-Haile et al. "Relaxation training reduces symptom reports and acid exposure in patients with gastroesophageal reflux disease." *Gastroenterology* 1994 Jul; 107(1): 61–69.

"The New Science of Siblings." *Time* magazine cover story, July 10, 2006.

Nilsson et al. "A comparison of intra-operative or postoperative exposure to music: a controlled trial of the effects on postoperative pain." *Anesthesia* 2003 Jul; 58 (7): 699–703.

Ornish et al. "Can lifestyle changes reverse coronary heart disease? The Lifestyle Heart Trial." *Lancet* 1990; 336: 129–33.

Ott et al. "Mindfulness meditation for oncology patients: a discussion and critical review." *Integrative Cancer Therapies* 2006 Jun; 5(2): 98.

Paul-Labrador et al. "Effects of a randomized control trial of transcendental meditation on components of the metabolic syndrome in subjects with coronary heart disease." *Archives of Internal Medicine* 2006 June; 166(11): 1218.

Penninx et al. "Minor and major depression and the risk of death in older persons." *Archives of General Psychiatry* 1999 Oct; 56(10): 889–95.

Peterson et al. "Pessimistic explanatory style is a risk factor for physical illness: a thirty-five-year longitudinal study." *Journal of Personality and Social Psychology* 1988 Jul; 55(1): 23–27.

Quintanilla et al. "Simple pre-surgical technique eases patient anxiety, saves money in recovery." Published 2004 Jun; online at http://www.imadulation.com/ blue-shield.htm.

Scheier. et al. "Optimism and rehospitalization after coronary artery bypass graft surgery." *Archives of Internal Medicine* 1999 Apr 26; 159(8): 829–35.

Schneider et al. "A randomized controlled trial of stress reduction for hypertension in older African Americans." *Hypertension* 1995 Nov; 26(5): 820.

"The Science of Meditation." *Time* magazine cover story, August 4, 2003.

Sephton et al. "Mindfulness meditation alleviates depressive symptoms in women with fibromyalgia: results of a randomized clinical trial." *Arthritis & Rheumatism* 2007 Feb 15; 57(1): 77.

Sesso et al. "Depression and the risk of coronary heart disease in the Normative Aging Study." *American Journal of Cardiology* 1998 Oct 1; 82(7): 851–56.

Shaw and Ehrlich. "Relaxation training as a treatment for chronic pain caused by ulcerative colitis." *Pain* 1987 Jun; 29(3): 287–93.

Smith et al. "Mindfulness-based stress reduction as supportive therapy in cancer care: systematic review." *Journal of Advanced Nursing* 2005 Nov; 52(3): 315.

Speca et al. "A randomized, wait-list controlled clinical trial: the effect of a mindfulness mediation stress-reduction program on mood and symptoms of stress in cancer outpatients." *Psychosomatic Medicine* 2000 Sep–Oct; 62(5): 613.

Suraway et al. "The effect of mindfulness training on mood and measures of fatigue, activity, and quality of life in patients with chronic fatigue syndrome." *Behavioral and Cognitive Psychotherapy* 2005; 33(1): 103.

Todaro, J.F. et al. "Effect of negative emotions on frequency of coronary heart disease (Normative Aging Study)." *American Journal of Cardiology* 2003 Oct 15; 92(8): 901–06.

Tusek, D.L. et al. "Guided imagery: a significant advance in the care of patients undergoing elective colorectal surgery." *Diseases of the Colon and Rectum.* 1997 Feb; 40(2): 172–78.

Weil, A. "Living Better Longer." *Time* magazine cover story, October 17, 2005.

Williams et al. "A randomized controlled trial of meditation and massage effects on quality of life in people with late-stage disease (HIV/AIDS)." *Journal of Palliative Medicine* 2005 Oct; 8(5): 939.

Winzelberg et al. "The effect of a meditation training in stress levels in secondary school teachers." *Stress Medicine* 1999; 15(2): 69.

Zamarra et al. "Usefulness of the transcendental meditation program in the treatment of patients with coronary artery disease." *American Journal of Cardiology* 1996 Apr; 77(10): 867.

Books

Ames, William L. "Emptiness and Quantum Theory." In *Buddhism and Science,* edited by B. Alan Wallace. New York: Columbia University Press, 2003.

Benson, Herbert. *The Relaxation Response* [1975]. New York: HarperCollins, 2000.

Bronowski, Jacob. *A Sense of the Future.* Cambridge, MA: MIT Press, 1978.

———. *The Ascent of Man* (BBC television series and book). Boston and Toronto: Little Brown, 1973.

Burns, Douglas M. *Buddhist Meditation and Depth Psychology.* Pariyatti Press, 1994.

Campbell, Don, comp. *Music: Physician for Times to Come* [1991]. Wheaton, IL: Quest Books, 2000.

Campbell, Don. *The Mozart Effect: Tapping the Power of Music to Heal* [1997]. New York: HarperCollins, 2001.

Campbell, T. Colin. *The China Study: The Most Comprehensive Study of Nutrition Ever Conducted and the Startling Implications for Diet, Weight Loss and Long-term Health.* Dallas, TX: BenBella Books, 2006.

Chopra, Deepak. *The Book of Secrets.* New York: Three Rivers Press, 2005.

Crick, Francis. *The Astonishing Hypothesis: The Scientific Search for the Soul.* New York and London: Touchstone, 1995.

Dalai Lama. *An Open Heart: Practicing Compassion in Everyday Life.* Boston, New York, and London: Little, Brown, 2001.

———. *Live in A Better Way.* New York: Penguin Compass, 2002.

———. *Stages of Meditation.* Ithaca, NY: Snow Lion Publications, 2001.

Dalai Lama and Howard Cutler. *The Art of Happiness.* New York: Simon & Schuster, 1998.

Damasio, Antonio. *Looking for Spinoza: Joy, Sorrow, and the Feeling Brain.* San Diego, New York, and London: Harcourt, Inc., 2003.

————. *The Feeling of What Happens: Body and Emotion in the Making of Consciousness.* San Diego, New York, and London: Harcourt Trade Publishers, 1999.

Dass, Ram. *Be Here Now.* San Anselmo, CA: Hanuman Foundation, 1971.

————. *Journey of Awakening: A Meditator's Guidebook.* New York: Bantam Books,1978.

————. *Still Here: Embracing Aging, Changing, and Dying.* New York: Riverhead Books, 2000.

Davidson, Richard J., ed. *Anxiety, Depression, and Emotion.* Oxford and New York: Oxford University Press, 2000.

De Spinoza, Benedict. *Ethics.* New York and London: Penguin Classics, 1996.

Dissanayake, Ellen. *Art and Intimacy: How the Arts Began.* Seattle and London: University of Washington Press, 2000.

Doidge, Norman. *The Brain That Changes Itself.* New York: Penguin Books, 2007.

Dyer, Wayne W. *Wisdom of the Ages.* New York: HarperCollins, 1998.

Easwaran, Eknath. *Meditation: A Simple Eight-Point Program for Translating Spiritual Ideas into Daily Life* [1978]. Tomales, CA: Nilgiri Press, 1991.

Edelman, Gerald. *Wider Than the Sky: The Phenomenal Gift of Consciousness.* New Haven, CT: Yale University Press, 2004.

Einstein, Albert. *Relativity: The Special and General Theory.* United Kingdom: Dodo Press, 1916.

Ekman, Paul. *Emotions Revealed* [2003]. New York: Holt Paperbacks, 2007.

Epstein, Mark. *Going to Pieces Without Falling Apart.* New York: Broadway Books, 1999.

————. *Thoughts Without a Thinker: Psychotherapy from a Buddhist Perspective.* New York: Basic Books, 1996.

Feynman, Richard. *The Feynman Lectures on Physics.* Indianapolis, IN: Addison-Wesley, 2005.

Franck, Frederick. *The Zen of Seeing: Seeing/Drawing As Meditation.* New York: Vintage Books, 1973.

Galin, David. "The Concepts 'Self,' 'Person,' and 'I' in Western Psychology and in Buddhism." In *Buddhism and Science,* edited by B. Alan Wallace. New York: Columbia University Press, 2003.

Gallwey, W. Timothy. *The Inner Game of Tennis* [1974]. New York: Random House, 1997.

Gethin, Rupert. *The Foundations of Buddhism.* New York and Oxford: Oxford University Press, 1998.

Goldberg, Elkhonon. *The Wisdom Paradox.* New York: Gotham Books, 2005.

Goldstein, Joseph. *Insight Meditation.* Boston and London: Shambhala Publications, 1993.

———. *One Dharma: The Emerging Western Buddhism.* New York: HarperCollins Publishers, 2002.

Goldstein, Rebecca. *Betraying Spinoza.* New York: Schocken Books, 2006.

Goleman, Daniel. *Destructive Emotions: How Can We Overcome Them? A Scientific Dialogue with the Dalai Lama.* New York: Bantam Dell, 2004.

———. *Social Intelligence.* New York: Bantam Dell, 2006.

Hesse, Hermann. *Journey to the East* [1932]. New York: Bantam Books, 1972.

———. *Narcissus and Goldmund* [1930]. New York: Farrar, Straus, and Giroux, 1968.

———. *Siddhartha* [1922]. New York: Bantam Classics, 1951.

———. *Steppenwolf* [1929]. New York: Picador, 2002.

Hut, Piet. "Life As a Laboratory." In *Buddhism and Science,* edited by B. Alan Wallace. New York: Columbia University Press, 2003.

Isaacson, Walter. *Einstein: His Life and Universe.* New York and London: Simon & Schuster, 2007.

Iyer, Pico. *The Open Road: The Global Journey of the Fourteenth Dalai Lama.* New York: Alfred A. Knopf, Inc., 2008.

Kabat-Zinn, Jon. *Coming to Our Senses.* New York: Hyperion, 2005.

———. *Full Catastrophe Living.* New York: Delta Trade Paperbacks, 1990.

———. *Wherever You Go There You Are.* New York: Hyperion, 1994.

Kerouac, Jack. *The Dharma Bums* [1958]. New York: Penguin Classics, 2006.

Klein, Shari and Neill Gibson. *What's Making You Angry?* Encinitas, CA: PuddleDancer Press, 2005.

Kornfield, Jack. *A Path with Heart.* New York: Bantam Books, 1993.

Kornfield, Jack, ed. *Teachings of the Buddha.* Boston and London: Shambhala, 1993, 1996.

LeDoux, Joseph. *Synaptic Self: How Our Brains Become Who We Are.* New York: Penguin Books, 2003.

Levitin, Daniel J. *This Is Your Brain on Music.* New York: Dutton, 2006.

Moses, Jeffrey. *Oneness: Great Principles Shared by All Religions* [1989]. New York: Ballantine Books, 2003.

Nhat Hanh, Thich. *Anger: Wisdom for Cooling the Flames.* New York: Riverhead Books, 2001.

———. *The Art of Power.* New York: HarperOne, 2007.

———. *Be Free Where You Are.* Berkeley, CA: Parallax Press, 2002.

———. *Call Me By My True Names.* Berkeley, CA: Parallax Press, 1999.

————. *Creating True Peace*. New York: Free Press, 2003.

————. *I Have Arrived, I Am Home: Celebrating 20 Years of Plum Village Life*. Berkeley, CA: Parallax Press, 2003.

————. *Interbeing*. Berkeley, CA: Parallax Press, 1998.

————. *Joyfully Together: The Art of Building a Harmonious Community*. Berkeley, CA: Parallax Press, 2003.

————. *The Long Road Turns to Joy: A Guide to Walking Meditation*. Berkeley, CA: Parallax Press, 1996.

————. *No Death, No Fear*. New York: Riverhead Books, 2002.

————. *Old Path White Clouds: Walking in the Footsteps of the Buddha*. Berkeley, CA: Parallax Press, 1991.

————. *Peace Is Every Step* [1991]. New York, Toronto, and London: Bantam Books, 1992.

————, comp. *Plum Village Chanting and Recitation Book*. Berkeley, CA: Parallax Press, 2000.

————. *Present Moment Wonderful Moment*. Berkeley, CA: Parallax Press, 1990.

————. *The Miracle of Mindfulness* [1976]. Boston: Beacon Press, 1987.

————. *The Sun My Heart*. Berkeley, CA: Parallax Press, 1988.

Nhat Hanh, Thich, trans. *The Sutra on Mindful Breathing*. Plum Village: Breath of the Buddha Retreat, June 2006.

Nhat Hanh, Thich. *Taming the Tiger Within: Meditations on Transforming Difficult Emotions*. New York: Riverhead Books, 2005.

————. *Touching the Earth*. Berkeley, CA: Parallax Press, 2004.

Ramachandran, V.S. *A Brief Tour of Human Consciousness*. New York: Pi Press, 2004.

Randall, Lisa. *Warped Passages, Unraveling the Mysteries of the Universe's Hidden Dimensions*. New York: Harper Perennial, 2006.

Restak, Richard. *Mozart's Brain and the Fighter Pilot: Unleashing Your Brain's Potential*. New York: Three Rivers Press, 2001.

Rosenberg, Marshall B. *Nonviolent Communication: A Language of Life*. Encinitas, CA: PuddleDancer Press, 2003.

Rosenberg, Marshall B. *Speak Peace in a World of Conflict*. Encinitas, CA: PuddleDancer Press, 2005.

————. *The Surprising Purpose of Anger*. Encinitas, CA: PuddleDancer Press, 2005.

Schwartz, Jeffrey and Sharon Begley. *The Mind and The Brain: Neuroplasticity and the Power of Mental Force*. New York: HarperCollins, 2002.

Steinbeck, John. *Cannery Row* [1945]. New York: Penguin Classics, 1994.

Suzuki, Daisetz T. *An Introduction to Zen Buddhism.* New York: Grove Press, 1964.

———. *Zen Buddhism: Selected Writings of D. T. Suzuki* [1956]. New York: Doubleday, 1996.

Tager, Mark, and Charles Jennings. *Whole Person Health Care.* Portland, OR: Victoria House, 1978.

Tolle, Eckhart. *A New Earth: Awakening to Your Life's Purpose.* New York: Dutton, 2005.

———. *The Power of Now.* Novato, CA: New World Library, 1997.

———. *Practicing the Power of Now.* Novato, CA: New World Library, 1999.

———. *Stillness Speaks.* Novato, CA: New World Library, 2003.

Vonnegut, Kurt. *A Man Without a Country.* New York, London, and Toronto: Seven Stories Press, 2005.

Wallace, B. Alan, ed. *Buddhism and Science: Breaking New Ground.* New York: Columbia University Press, 2003.

Watts, Alan. *Become What You Are.* Boston and London: Shambhala, 1995.

———. *The Book: On the Taboo Against Knowing Who You Are* [1966]. New York: Vintage Books, 1989.

———. *The Way of Zen.* New York: Vintage Books, 1957.

Watts, Alan, and Mark Watts. *Zen: The Supreme Experience.* London: Vega, 2002.

Weil, Andrew. *Healthy Aging.* New York: Alfred A. Knopf, 2005.

Weinstein, Bruce. *Life Principles.* Cincinnati, OH: Emmis Books, 2005.

Wordsworth, William, and Samuel Coleridge. *Lyrical Ballads* [1798]. New York: Penguin Classics, 2007.

World Peace Prayer Society. *May Peace Prevail on Earth.* www.worldpeace.org.

Yogananda, Paramahansa. *Autobiography of a Yogi.* New York: The Philosophical Library, 1946.

———. *Scientific Healing Affirmations: Theory and Practice of Concentration* [1958]. Los Angeles: Self Realization Fellowship, 1990.

Audio CDs and Audiotapes

Bennett, Tony. "Smile" and "Put on a Happy Face" on *Tony Bennett Duets: An American Classic.* Sony, 2006.

Armstrong, Louis. *What a Wonderful World.* Verve, 1996.

Campbell, Don, comp. *Heal Yourself with Sound and Music.* Boulder, CO: Sounds True, 2000.

————. *Music for the Mozart Effect* (Vol 1). Spring Hill, 1998.

Cheatham, Jeannie and Jimmy. *Blues and the Boogie Masters.* Concord Jazz, 1993.

Kabat-Zinn, Jon. *Guided Mindfulness Meditation.* Boulder, CO: Sounds True, 2002.

————. *Mindfulness Meditation.* New York: Simon & Schuster, 1995.

Khong, Chan. *Total Relaxation and Touching of the Earth.* Plum Village Production. Berkeley, CA: Parallax Press, 2003.

Nhat Hanh, Thich. Dharma talks given at Deer Park Monastery, Winter Retreat. Deer Park Production, Berkeley, CA: Parallax Press, 2004.

————. Dharma talks given at Plum Village Monastery, Spring Retreat. Plum Village Production. Berkeley, CA: Parallax Press, 2006.

————. *The Art of Mindful Living.* Boulder, CO: Sounds True, 2000.

Nhat Hanh, Thich and Plum Village. *A Basket of Plums.* United Buddhist Church. Berkeley, CA: Parallax Press.

Taylor, James. "Secret O' Life" on *James Taylor (Live).* Country Road Music, 1993.

Watts, Alan. *Alan Watts Teaches Meditation.* Los Angeles: Audio Renaissance Tapes, 1973, 1992 by Electronic University.

Weiss, Gabriel. *Mindful.* Vista, CA: self-produced, 2003.

————. *Watering the Seeds.* Vista, CA: self-produced, 2005.

————. *Teaching Meditation.* Laguna Beach, CA: Basic Health Publications, 2008.

Videotapes, Films, and DVDs

Blumer, Ronald, and Muffie Meyer. *The New Medicine* (PBS special). Middlemarch Films, 2006.

Keep, Lennlee. *The Brain Fitness Program* (PBS special). Arlington, VA: Public Broadcasting Service, 2008.

Penn, Gregory. *Vipassana Meditation.* Carmel, CA: Aspire!, 1999.

Dass, Ram. *Fierce Grace.* Zeitgeist Films Ltd., [2001], 2003.

Weiss, Gabriel [Robert Alan]. *Protein Synthesis: An Epic on the Cellular Level.* Filmed at Palo Alto, CA: Stanford University, 1971, produced by The Senses Bureau, Department of Chemistry, University of California, San Diego. Distributed with explanatory booklet by Harper & Row Publishers, Media Division, 1971.

Publishing
and Photo Credits

The author and publisher would like to thank the following for their kind permission to reproduce their photographs and material from their books.

Publishing Credits

Excerpts from *The Ascent of Man* by Jacob Bronowski, copyright © 1973 by Jacob Bronowski, reprinted courtesy of Little, Brown & Co.

Excerpt from *Creating True Peace* by Thich Nhat Hanh, copyright © 2003 by The Venerable Thich Nhat Hanh, reprinted with permission of The Free Press, a Division of Simon & Schuster Adult Publishing Group. All rights reserved.

Excerpts from Dharma talks given by Thich Nhat Hanh at Plum Village Monastery (audio CD), Spring Retreat, 2006, used with permission of Parallax Press, Berkeley, CA; www.parallax.org.

Excerpts from Dharma talks given by Thich Nhat Hanh at Deer Park Monastery (audio CD), Winter Retreat, 2004, with permission of Parallax Press, Berkeley, CA; www-parallax.org.

"Too Many Goodbyes" by Jeannie Cheatham, published by Jim Jean Music, used with permission of Jeannie Cheatham.

Excerpts from *The Long Road Turns to Joy: A Guide to Walking Meditation* by Thich Nhat Hanh, 1996, used with permission of Parallax Press, Berkeley, CA; www.parallax.org.

Excerpts from *The Mind and the Brain* by Jeffrey Schwartz and Sharon Begley, copyright © 2002 by Jeffrey Schwartz and Sharon Begley, reprinted courtesy of Harper-Collins Publishers.

Excerpts from *Old Path White Clouds: Walking in the Footsteps of the Buddha* by Thich Nhat Hanh, 1991, used with permission of Parallax Press, Berkeley, CA; www.parallax.org.

Excerpts from *Plum Village Chanting and Recitation Book* compiled by Thich Nhat Hanh, 2000, used with permission of Parallax Press, Berkeley, CA; www. parallax.org.

Excerpts from *Present Moment Wonderful Moment* by Thich Nhat Hanh, 1990, used with permission of Parallax Press, Berkeley, CA; www.parallax.org.

"Too Many Goodbyes" by Jeannie Cheatham, published by Jim Jean Music, used with permission of Jeannie Cheatham.

Excerpts from *The Wisdom Paradox* by Elkhonon Goldberg, copyright © 2005 by Elkhonon Goldberg, used by permission of Gotham Books, an imprint of Penguin Group (USA), Inc.

Photo Credits

Figure 1. Buddha at Wat Pho in Bangkok; courtesy of Heidi Mokrzycki.

Figure 2. Land's End Labyrinth; courtesy of author.

Figure 3. Zen Rock Garden; courtesy of author.

Figure 4. Sanskrit symbol of OM; courtesy of Rosemary KimBal.

Figure 5. *Protein Synthesis;* courtesy of author.

Figure 6. Anatomy of the brain. Brain image courtesy of H.O.P.E.S. Project (Huntington's Outreach Project for Education at Stanford), Stanford University; www.stanford.edu/group/hopes.

Gallery Credits

Plate 1. Stained glass window in Ocean of Peace Meditation Hall; courtesy of author.

Plate 2. Equanimity in nature; courtesy of author.

Plate 3. Lotus blossom; courtesy of author.

Plate 4. *I Have Arrived* by Thich Nhat Hanh; courtesy of author.

Plate 5. *Courage;* courtesy of Rosemary KimBal.

Plate 6. Buddha statue at Deer Park Monastery; courtesy of author.

Plate 7. Ancient Greek statue of Asclepius; courtesy of author.

Plate 8. Bamboo flute being played by Adrienne Nims; courtesy of Adrienne Nims (www.AdrienneNims.com).

Plate 9. Tea house at Japanese Tea Garden; courtesy of author.

Plate 10. Teapot and bowl with colored clay; courtesy of Lana Wilson.

Index

About the Author

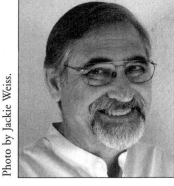

Photo by Jackie Weiss.

Gabriel S. Weiss, MD, is a graduate of Stanford University Medical School. As an internal medicine physician in general medical practice for the last thirty years, he has medical offices in both Oceanside and San Marcos, California. Dr. Weiss is a member of the active medical staff of Tri-City Medical Center in Oceanside, where he has also previously served as Chief of Internal Medicine and Chairman of the Department of Medicine.

He has actively practiced meditation for thirty-seven years. As founder and Medical Director of the Asclepius Wellness Center in Oceanside, he has taught meditation classes for many years. Also for years he has been a lay member of the sangha at Deer Park Monastery in Escondido, California, where he has practiced Zen meditation in the tradition of Zen master Thich Nhat Hanh.

Gabriel Weiss also plays jazz trumpet, and as a music composer and bandleader has produced six jazz and music therapy audio CDs, the latest of which is entitled *Watering the Seeds*. He has written and directed four educational movies, one of which, *Protein Synthesis: An Epic On the Cellular Level,* has become a "cult classic" in high school and college biology classes across the United States.

Dr. Weiss and his wife Jackie, who is a full-time high school dance teacher, live in Vista, California. They have two grown children, Shenandoah and Jasmine.

ABOUT THE ILLUSTRATOR

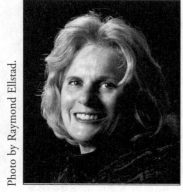

Photo by Raymond Ellstad.

Rosemary KimBal is an accomplished artist and illustrator with over thirty years of experience, specializing in contemporary Zen painting. Her artistic career began in 1971 when she was studying Zen and attended meditation sessions at the Tassajara Zen Mountain Center in the central coastal mountains of California. KimBal is influential in national and international circles that celebrate the ancient art of Zen painting. Using a free and spontaneous technique, her painting styles range from the traditional to the abstract. KimBal has illustrated ten other published books. Her art also includes works on rice paper, canvas, fabric, scrolls, note cards, clay, ceramic tile, film and theatrical scenic design.

Art critic Pat Stein wrote about Rosemary KimBal: "Once the brush is dipped into the ink, the stroke is executed with the speed of a pelican swooping into the surf for a fish, but the mental energy has already been marshaled and the intent is clear."

Watching her work, one realizes that the preparation of the artist's materials is a mindful process, a form of meditation. She selects the correct brush for the image in mind, dips into the ink and in flashing strokes, the subject blooms upon the surface. Her "dancing brush" has caught the essence of her subject.

Rosemary KimBal's work has been shown in galleries throughout the United States, Canada, and Taiwan. She represented "Zen Painting in America" at the Ronin Gallery in New York City in 1999. KimBal was selected by General Electric to teach the Creativity Workshop at the Fortune Most Powerful Women's Summit held in 2005, and again for General Electric in 2006.

Rosemary lives with her husband Raymond Ellstad, who is a photographer, in Cardiff-by-the-Sea, California. More information about her Dancing Brush Studios can be found at the following website: www.dancingbrush.com.